Trauma-Informed and Embodied
Approaches to Body Dysmorphic Disorder

By the same author

The Parents' Guide to Body Dysmorphic Disorder
How to Support Your Child, Teen or Young Adult
Nicole Schnackenberg, Benedetta Monzani and Amita Jassi
Foreword by Rob Willson and David Veale
ISBN 978 1 78775 113 2
eISBN 978 1 78775 114 9

Of related interest

Appearance Anxiety
A Guide to Understanding Body Dysmorphic Disorder
for Young People, Families and Professionals
*National and Specialist OCD, BDD and Related
Disorders Service, Maudsley Hospital*
ISBN 978 1 78592 456 9
eISBN 978 1 78450 832 6

Counselling Skills for Working with Shame
Christiane Sanderson
ISBN 978 1 84905 562 8
eISBN 978 1 78450 001 6

Confronting Shame
How to Understand Your Shame and Gain Inner Freedom
Ilse Sand
ISBN 978 1 83997 140 2
eISBN 978 1 83997 141 9

Trauma-Sensitive Yoga
Dagmar Härle
Foreword by David Emerson
ISBN 978 1 84819 346 8
eISBN 978 0 85701 301 9

Trauma-Informed and Embodied Approaches to Body Dysmorphic Disorder

Edited by **Nicole Schnackenberg**

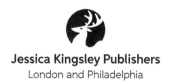

Jessica Kingsley Publishers
London and Philadelphia

First published in Great Britain in 2023 by Jessica Kingsley Publishers
An imprint of John Murray Press

1

A CIP catalogue record for this title is available from the
British Library and the Library of Congress

ISBN 978 1 83997 686 5
eISBN 978 1 83997 687 2

Printed and bound by CPI Group (UK) Ltd, Croydon, CR0 4YY

Jessica Kingsley Publishers' policy is to use papers that are natural,
renewable and recyclable products and made from wood grown in
sustainable forests. The logging and manufacturing processes are expected
to conform to the environmental regulations of the country of origin.

Jessica Kingsley Publishers
Carmelite House
50 Victoria Embankment
London EC4Y 0DZ

www.jkp.com

John Murray Press
Part of Hodder & Stoughton Limited
An Hachette UK Company

Contents

Introduction

What Is BDD and How Might Trauma-Informed, Embodied Approaches Help?

――――――

NICOLE SCHNACKENBERG

One's perception of, and relationship with, one's physical body can change across the lifespan including through patterns of wellness and illness, and life changes and stages like adolescence, pregnancy, menopause and ageing. It may even change day to day; or, for some people, from moment to moment.

Many people experience some level of dissatisfaction with the appearance of their body at some point during their lifespan. For some this will be fleeting while for others it will be pervasive and long-lasting. Body image struggles exist on a continuum with mild body image dissatisfaction on one end and clinical levels of distress, such as in the form of diagnoses like eating disorders and body dysmorphic disorder (BDD), on the other.

BDD is a lesser known and understood appearance-focused mental health diagnosis that most typically begins in adolescence, although it can affect people of, and emerge at, any age. BDD is characterised by a distressing preoccupation with perceived appearance defect(s) or flaw(s) that are either not visible to the outside eye or are perceived by the outside eye as simply part of normal human variation. The diagnostic criteria for BDD cite a distressing preoccupation which consumes the person for at least an hour a day. The reality, however, for many people living with BDD is that their distressing preoccupation consumes much of their day (and sometimes night), or indeed is all they can think about. The distressing preoccupation with the perceived appearance defect or flaw may prevent engagement in activities of daily living like going to school or work, interacting socially and even leaving the house.

BDD is estimated to affect 2–3 per cent of the population, making it more common than better-understood mental health struggles such as anorexia. Despite its relatively high prevalence rate, there appears to be less understanding of, and support for, BDD than many other mental health struggles. This may, in part, be because research into BDD only started in earnest in the 1970s; and BDD has been researched considerably less than many other mental health struggles. The significant levels of shame surrounding BDD may also have something to do with it, which can prevent people from seeking help and being forthright about their struggles. The many assumptions surrounding BDD are part of this story, including misconceptions that BDD is related to vanity in some way. In fact, people struggling with BDD are not vain in any sense. Rather, they are yearning and striving to have a physical appearance they feel will not repulse, and ignite rejection by, others.

BDD is classified under the umbrella of 'Obsessive Compulsive and Related Disorders' in the *Diagnostic and Statistical Manual of Mental Disorders* (DSM-V) and the *International Classification of Diseases* (ICD-11). This is due to the main preoccupation with the appearance being obsessional in nature. This typically includes repetitive behaviours like touching the perceived defect and compulsive checking of the appearance in the mirror (or compulsive avoidance of the mirror; or oscillation between checking and avoiding); and avoidance behaviours like avoiding social situations and covering up the perceived defect with make-up, clothing etc.

People with a diagnosis of BDD are typically dissatisfied with around three body parts at any one time, with one usually causing the most distress. They can become preoccupied with their perceived defects to such an extent that they experience significant emotional distress, including feelings of depression, anxiety and suicidality. In fact, BDD has one of the highest suicide rates associated with any mental health diagnosis (Phillips et al., 2005; Veale et al., 2016).

People are often surprised to learn that BDD affects people who identify as males and females almost equally. Research which includes the experiences of those who identify as gender non-binary is yet to be undertaken. In terms of muscle dysmorphia, a sub-type of BDD, however, more people who identify as males receive this diagnosis than those who identify as females. People diagnosed with muscle dysmorphia experience distress that their body build is too small or insufficiently muscular. They may spend extended time periods in the gym, and follow a strict, high-protein diet. They may also take steroids, particularly anabolic androgenic steroids. These substances, of course, come with health-related dangers of their own.

Despite its relatively high prevalence rate, a lot of people (including some medical and mental health professionals) have not heard of BDD nor received any training in its recognition or treatment. You are not alone, therefore, if you are a clinician or therapist who has not come across the term 'BDD' before and/or are – or have met – a person who has had their experience of BDD ignored or minimised. It is my hope, and the shared hope of the contributing authors, that this book will both validate and help you to better understand the experience of BDD and how to support those struggling.

The National Institute for Clinical Excellence (NICE) Guidelines in the UK recommend Cognitive Behavioural Therapy (CBT) with Exposure Response Prevention (ERP) for BDD, alongside selective serotonin reuptake inhibitors (SSRIs – a class of anti-depressant medication). Indeed, the largest evidence base in terms of treatment for BDD has thus far been for BDD-specific CBT which includes the ERP element. Far less research has been conducted into modalities outside of the cognitive behavioural realm, although the evidence base is steadily growing. Importantly, both empirical research and anecdotal accounts are increasingly highlighting the necessity of exploring trauma (particularly developmental trauma), shame, felt sense of identity and the paucity of self-compassion in those experiencing BDD. The focus of this book will be on considering how trauma-informed, embodied practices may be beneficial, which comprise approaches sitting outside of the CBT paradigm.

It is important to be clear that, of course, no treatment modality or practice should or could claim to be a complete 'cure all' for BDD and associated struggles. As we have considered, research into approaches outside of CBT for people struggling with BDD is very much in its infancy. Therefore, some of the research drawn upon in the chapters of this book has been conducted with people experiencing associated struggles like anxiety, depression, eating difficulties, generalised body image distress and post-traumatic stress. The suggestion, rather (which is backed up by a growing body of empirical research) is that the practices and approaches contained within this book may be supportive in relation to many aspects of the experience of BDD including aiding in the soothing and regulation of the nervous system; reducing rumination and compulsive behaviours; increasing interoceptive awareness; reducing shame; increasing capacity for self-compassion; and offering a window into a sense of self beyond the thoughts and the physical body.

How Do I Know If My Client Is Struggling with BDD?

Only a trained health professional can make a clinical diagnosis of BDD. Sometimes, people will use online screening tools to determine whether BDD may be part of their experience. They may then print these out to share with their GP (general practitioner), psychiatrist etc. Online versions of two widely used, evidence-based tools, the COPS (Cosmetic Procedure Screening) and the Appearance Anxiety Inventory, are freely available on the BDD Foundation website. Therapists may also choose to use these tools with their clients to explore their experiences; or to refer to them if they suspect they may be supporting someone for whom BDD is part of their experience.

It is important to note that there are people who self-identify as experiencing BDD without having a formal diagnosis. Furthermore, while a diagnosis can be validating for some people, others may prefer to seek and proceed with therapy without a diagnosis of BDD. In an ideal world, mental health diagnoses would not hold the key to unlocking funding for treatment, though this unfortunately continues to be the case in many geographical areas across the globe. Regardless, it is beneficial to come alongside your client's conceptualisation of their distress, using the language they feel most comfortable with to describe and make sense of their struggles. This will include using the term 'BDD' with some clients and using other language, like 'appearance-focused distress', with others. The term 'BDD' is used throughout this book for ease of reading, in full awareness of the debate around the questionable validity of psychiatric diagnoses and with the utmost respect for other conceptualisations and ways of languaging human suffering of this kind.

Why Do People Struggle with BDD?

It is unclear precisely why some people experience a distressing and pervasive preoccupation with an aspect or aspects of their appearance. What is becoming increasingly evident, however, is that BDD is underpinned by a complex array of inter-linking factors. These include: biological factors (such as differences in brain neurochemistry); evolutionary factors (including social belongingness/rejection and abandonment sensitivity); life experience factors (including trauma, such as developmental/relational trauma and/or appearance-focused bullying and teasing in childhood); visual processing differences (a propensity to process visual information locally rather than globally, and to focus on detail as opposed to the 'big picture'); an anxious and/or perfectionistic temperament; pervasive feelings of shame and/or pre-existing low self-esteem/poor self-concept; and a fragmented sense of self.

People with BDD pin their identity and self-worth onto their appearance, 'blaming' any feelings of shame, sense of unlovability, 'not-good-enoughness', anxiety and sense of isolation they feel on the way they look. They then desperately hold on to the belief that once their appearance defect is 'fixed' they will become a lovable, safe, 'good enough' and contented human being. However, once one aspect of the appearance is 'fixed' or 'improved' within the context of BDD, the appearance focus tends to move on to another aspect of the appearance. This is hardly surprising given that the root of BDD has nothing to do with appearance defects at all and is not, therefore, going to be 'solved' by 'fixing' the appearance. Rather, BDD is composed of feelings of shame, misplaced identity and low self-worth, typically in the context of immensely painful and emotionally overwhelming life experiences, particularly of relational trauma. Throughout this book we will explore the underlying shame and low self-worth underpinning BDD and consider how trauma-informed, embodied practices may be helpful to those struggling.

Is the Media to Blame?

BDD is sometimes blamed on the media, including (and perhaps especially) on social media. It is true that the mainstream media bombards us with hundreds if not thousands of images each day, many of which display similar and narrow 'homogenous' gendered body types. It is also true that social media can display and perpetuate unrealistic appearance 'ideals' and prompt comparisons and aspirations in relation to such 'ideals'. It would also seem that the younger generation are almost socially expected to be on social media and to use it as a way of making and maintaining a relational connection with others.

However, BDD is not caused by the media, although it may rarely do little to help the situation. If the media directly caused BDD then all consumers of the media would struggle with BDD, and it wouldn't have been identified as long ago as in 1891 – referred to at the time as dysmorphophobia.

Common Diagnoses which Overlap with BDD

Psychiatric diagnoses are made by psychiatrists and other health professionals who execute a judgment based on a list of observable behaviours. Given the subjective nature of such an approach, it is common for people experiencing BDD (and indeed other mental health struggles) to receive other diagnoses before, after and even at the same time as their diagnosis of BDD as many of the behaviours are similar across diagnoses. Some of the most common diagnoses which overlap with BDD include eating disorders, obsessive compulsive disorder (OCD), skin picking disorder (dermatillomania/excoriation), hair pulling disorder (trichotillomania), depression, anxiety (particularly social anxiety) and substance misuse disorder.

Eating Disorders

Eating disorders are common occurrences alongside BDD. Some of the eating-related diagnoses associated with BDD are anorexia, bulimia, orthorexia, binge-eating disorder and OSFED (otherwise specified feeding and eating disorder). Eating disorders and BDD, however, sit in separate diagnostic categories. If the focus of distress is on the overall weight and shape of the body, a diagnosis of an eating disorder is more likely to be made than a diagnosis of BDD. However, if any food restriction or food-related behaviours taking place are with the aim of altering a specific body part such as the shape of the face, a diagnosis of BDD may be given.

These experiences, however, are not as cut and dried as the clinical diagnostic manuals would have us believe. Many people diagnosed with BDD also have symptoms of an eating disorder and may experience both diagnoses. Most commonly, people experiencing BDD may cut out certain foods or food groups with the aim of altering, or preventing changes to, the body part which is the focus of their distress. For example, a person may avoid foods containing oil in an attempt to prevent skin blemishes, or only eat blandly coloured foods to prevent the teeth from becoming stained. Some people might attempt to lose weight, but perhaps in order to change a particular aspect of their appearance, e.g. to make the face appear thinner, rather than hoping to change the overall weight and shape of the body.

Nutritional restriction can have a range of devastating physiological ramifications including low blood pressure, blood sugar level imbalances, electrolyte imbalances, reduced bone density, heartbeat arrhythmias, digestive issues and organs struggling to carry out their functions optimally, to name just a few possibilities. Some of these physiological manifestations can be potentially fatal. When working with people experiencing BDD who are chronically restricting their nutritional intake, therefore, regardless of whether or not they are classified as underweight, an assessment by a medical doctor is of paramount importance.

Obsessive Compulsive Disorder

OCD comes under the same umbrella as BDD in the DSM-V and the ICD-11, namely under 'Obsessive Compulsive and Related Disorders'. This is because OCD and BDD share many features including compulsive and obsessive behaviours and thoughts. The main difference is that in BDD the compulsions and obsessions are directly related to perceived defects in the appearance. Another difference is that shame does not tend to underpin OCD in the way it pervasively and fundamentally underlies and fuels BDD.

OCD can cause extremely high levels of distress and impact negatively on daily functioning. Colloquial narratives around people 'being a bit OCD' because they like to clean their house regularly, for example, sadly seem to have diminished the seriousness of OCD in many peoples' minds and led to a great deal of misunderstanding.

OCD is characterised by intensely negative, repetitive and intrusive thoughts, combined with chronic feelings of danger or doubt (obsessions). In order to quieten the thoughts or alleviate the anxiety, the person will often repeat actions again and again (compulsions). Embodied, trauma-informed practices are replete with tools for soothing anxiety and regulating the nervous system, which we will explore in more detail in the coming chapters of this book.

Skin Picking Disorder (Dermatillomania/Excoriation) and Hair Pulling Disorder (Trichotillomania)

Skin picking disorder and hair pulling disorder are body-focused repetitive behaviours which also come under the umbrella of 'Obsessive Compulsive and Related Disorders' in the diagnostic manuals of mental disorders. Skin picking disorder is characterised by repeatedly picking at one's skin resulting in skin lesions and causing significant disruptions in a person's life. It also extends to pulling, scraping and biting both healthy and damaged skin from various parts of the body, including hands, fingers, arms and legs, though most often on the face. Due to intense feelings of shame, people may attempt to cover up any skin lesions with clothing, make-up or using other means, similarly to the way in which people with BDD may cover up (camouflage) aspects of their appearance in order to conceal their perceived defect(s) and/or flaw(s).

People may compulsively pick at their skin for a number of reasons; it can be an attempt to soothe feelings of nervous system dysregulation/ anxiety and/or be an attempt to harm the self. Skin picking can also be associated with perfectionism, e.g. picking at the skin in an attempt to make it 'flat' or 'smooth', often linked with excessive grooming. Within the experience of BDD, skin picking most typically occurs in an attempt to remove blemishes and/or soothe uncomfortable feelings such as anxiety, shame and low mood.

Hair pulling disorder is characterised by recurrent, irresistible urges to pull the hair out from the scalp, eyebrows or other areas of the body, despite trying to stop. This can leave bald patches, which may cause significant distress and interfere with daily functioning. Again, people may try to cover up these bald patches due to feelings of shame, perhaps using hats, head scarves, baggy clothing etc.

You will find numerous trauma-informed, embodied practices relevant to supporting skin picking and hair pulling experiences throughout this book.

Depression and Anxiety

Clinical levels of depression and anxiety (including social anxiety) are a common experience for people with a diagnosis of BDD. Approaches for supporting clients experiencing anxiety and depression are peppered throughout this book as they are so closely linked with the experience of BDD.

Substance Misuse

A proportion of people diagnosed with BDD will also be diagnosed with a substance misuse disorder. Substances like alcohol and non-prescription drugs are most typically used by people experiencing BDD to soothe feelings of anxiety, particularly social anxiety as explored in more detail by

Tristan Keller in Chapter 9. It is important to note that embodied practices and non-prescription drugs/alcohol are not an ideal or beneficial
combination: it is important to encourage and support clients to come
to any therapeutic sessions in a sober state.

What Help/Treatment Is Available to People with BDD?

As we touched upon at the beginning of this Introduction, many people have not heard of BDD despite its high prevalence rate relative to
better-known/understood mental health struggles. Awareness is gradually increasing, however, which will hopefully lead to people receiving
support in a timelier manner.

As we explored at the beginning of this Introduction, the treatment
recommended by NICE for people diagnosed with BDD in the UK is
BDD-specific CBT with ERP, often accompanied with a high dose of SSRIs
(a kind of antidepressant medication). Other approaches – including
those contained within this book (such as Compassion Focused Therapy)
have shown promise with people struggling with BDD.

Many people with BDD report finding attendance at online and
in-person BDD-specific support groups significantly helpful, as they
tend to facilitate a felt sense of genuine understanding from others and
a reduction in feelings of loneliness and isolation. Online groups can
feel more accessible for people severely struggling, as the camera can be
turned off and the person may simply listen in if that is what helps them
the most. Numerous groups are run by both the BDD Foundation and
OCD Action in the UK, and more details can be found on the websites
of each organisation.

What Do We Mean by Trauma-Informed, Embodied Approaches?

Trauma-informed practices explicitly consider, acknowledge and address
the role trauma and traumatic stress play in a person's life. To qualify as
being trauma-informed, an approach or system of care should demonstrate an understanding of the complexity of trauma and a recognition
of it as a phenomenon that is both socio-political and interpersonal
(occurring between people as opposed to being something that happens
'inside' a person in isolation). When considering the impact trauma has
played in a person's life, the Power Threat Meaning Framework (PTFM)
(Johnstone et al., 2018) advocates closely considering:

- *Power*: How power has operated in a person's life.

- *Threat*: What threat this power has posed to them.

- *Meaning*: What meaning they have made of this threat.

In the context of BDD, these are vital questions to explore as part of any therapeutic modality, considering, as part of these three core PTFM questions, the Social GGRRAAACCEEESSS (SG) (Burnham, 2018): *Gender, Geography, Race, Religion, Age, Ability, Appearance, Culture, Class/Caste, Education, Employment, Ethnicity, Spirituality, Sexuality* and *Sexual Orientation*. Taking one of these 'Graces' as an example, namely race, we might explore with our clients:

- Any experience of power differentials, past and present, in relation to race, including both implicit and explicit messages about who holds power in the family/community etc. in relation to cultural background, colour of the skin etc.

- If, when and how they have experienced any threat in relation to their race.

- What meaning they have made from any racially related threats they have experienced, including meanings made about their felt sense of identity, appearance and place in their families, communities, workplace etc.

What Can Trauma-Informed, Embodied Approaches Offer to People Struggling with BDD?

This book advocates and offers embodied practices which are trauma-informed. Embodied practices pay attention to the sensations in the body as avenues towards understanding, awareness, self-regulation, empowerment and healing. There is a growing body of scientific research indicating the efficacy of trauma-informed, embodied practices for a range of experiences related to BDD. For example:

- Reduction in feelings of anxiety and depression (e.g. D'Alessio et al., 2020; Saeed, Cunningham & Bloch, 2019).

- Increased interoceptive awareness (the lived experience of the body from the inside) (e.g. Neukirch, Reid & Shires, 2019).

- Improved nervous system regulation and emotional regulation (e.g. Jung & Lee, 2021; Lucas et al., 2018).

- Reduction in behaviours associated with diagnoses of eating struggles (e.g. Hafid & Kerna, 2019; Rizzuto et al., 2021).

- Reduction in compulsions and obsessions (e.g. Leeuwerik, Cavanagh & Strauss, 2020; Mehta et al., 2020).

- Reduction in addictive behaviours (e.g. Galantino et al., 2021).

- Increased feelings of self-compassion (e.g. Frostadottir & Dorjee, 2019).

Trauma-informed, embodied practices can also offer experiences of the self (which we could call the core self, original self or true self) beyond the physical body and appearance. Such experiences can invite a sense of spaciousness and peacefulness around one's felt sense of identity, and remind and reconnect a person with their values. As we will explore throughout this book, one's felt sense of identity is a central aspect of the experience of BDD, typically a felt sense of self saturated in shame. Thus, at their best, the approaches offered throughout this book involve an exploration and soothing of shame, and reconnect a person with their innate lovability.

With this in mind, the book begins with a personal account of BDD by Anna, an expert-by-lived-experience, who shares how yoga, meditation and Eye Movement Desensitisation and Reprocessing (EMDR) therapy were particularly supportive in her journey with BDD. We then move on to hearing from Arie, Founder and Director of the BDD Clinic in Los Angeles, about how emotional developmental trauma can be an aspect underpinning the experience of BDD, laying the foundation stone for our consideration of trauma-informed, embodied approaches throughout the rest of the book. In Chapter 3 doctoral researcher and clinician Natalie considers BDD in the context of intimate relationships, exploring how therapists can support their clients to both acknowledge and work with the relational suffering so characteristic of the experience of BDD. In Chapter 4, we return to hearing directly from an expert-by-lived-experience (and psychologist), Alex, who reflects on how artwork has been a conduit for his eye for detail and aesthetic proclivities. Chapter 5 is an offering by myself, delving into some neuroscientific insights including how this knowledge, especially about the right and left hemispheres of the brain, can be practically drawn upon in the therapeutic space.

Jo offers us some insights into how movement, particularly yoga, has been supportive in her journey with BDD in Chapter 6 before we move on to hearing from family therapist Jill in Chapter 7, who also uses yoga alongside non-violent resistance in her work. We shift direction slightly in Chapter 8, wherein I take us on an exploration of the nervous system including aspects of Polyvagal Theory in the context of BDD, which leads us nicely into Tristan's consideration of the importance of nutrition, including its impact on the nervous system, in Chapter 9.

Acceptance and Commitment Therapy principles are the focus of psychologist Sarah's contribution in Chapter 10, which flows into Chapter 11 wherein psychotherapist Rosa offers some ways of using Compassion Focused Therapy approaches with clients. As we come to the end of the book, we return to EMDR in Chapter 12, this time from the perspective of Beverley, an EMDR therapist who uses it to poignant effect with clients experiencing BDD.

Chapter 13 continues and expands upon the theme of self-compassion, written by myself and my husband, Joachim, and outlining how we have used the Voice Dialogue approach in the context of BDD, including to support clients in viewing their BDD as a frightened and protective aspect of the self. Therapist and Chair of the BDD Foundation, Rob, also picks up the theme of compassion in Chapter 14, this time in the context of an approach called Imagery Rescripting, before Tristan's final chapter on supporting authenticity and a felt sense of the true self in those experiencing BDD. Mental health activist and expert-by-lived-experience James and I then close the book with some final reflections, which we hope will offer the reader some parting food for thought and invite an appetite for further reading and exploration into trauma-informed and embodied approaches for BDD.

References

Burnham, J. (2018). Developments in social GGRRAAACCEEESSS: Visible–invisible and voiced–unvoiced 1. In I. B. Krause (ed.), *Culture and reflexivity in systemic psychotherapy* (pp. 139–160). Routledge.

D'Alessio, L., Korman, G. P., Sarudiansky, M., Guelman, L. R., Scévola, L., Pastore, A., ... & Roldán, E. J. (2020). Reducing allostatic load in depression and anxiety disorders: Physical activity and yoga practice as add-on therapies. *Frontiers in Psychiatry, 11*, 501.

Frostadottir, A. D., & Dorjee, D. (2019). Effects of mindfulness based cognitive therapy (MBCT) and Compassion Focused Therapy (CFT) on symptom change, mindfulness, self-compassion, and rumination in clients with depression, anxiety, and stress. *Frontiers in Psychology, 10*, 1099.

Galantino, M. L., Turetzkin, S., Lawlor, S., Jones, L., & Brooks, J. C. (2021). Community-based yoga for women undergoing substance use disorder treatment: A descriptive study. *International Journal of Yoga, 14*(1), 50.

Hafid, A., & Kerna, N. A. (2019). Adjunct application of mindfulness-based stress reduction in anorexia nervosa. *EC Psychology and Psychiatry, 8*(12), 1–6.

Johnstone, L., Boyle, M., Cromby, J., Dillon, J., Harper, D., Kinderman, P., & Read, J. (2018). *The power threat meaning framework: Towards the identification of patterns in emotional distress, unusual experiences and troubled or troubling behaviour, as an alternative to functional psychiatric diagnosis.* British Psychological Society.

Jung, M., & Lee, M. (2021). The effect of a mindfulness-based education program on brain waves and the autonomic nervous system in university students. *Healthcare, 9*(11), 1606.

Leeuwerik, T., Cavanagh, K., & Strauss, C. (2020). The association of trait mindfulness and self-compassion with obsessive-compulsive disorder symptoms: Results from a large survey with treatment-seeking adults. *Cognitive Therapy and Research, 44*(1), 120–135.

Lucas, A. R., Klepin, H. D., Porges, S. W., & Rejeski, W. J. (2018). Mindfulness-based movement: A polyvagal perspective. *Integrative Cancer Therapies, 17*(1), 5–15.

Mehta, K., Mehta, S., Chalana, H., Singh, H., & Thaman, R. G. (2020). Effectiveness of Rajyoga meditation as an adjunct to first-line treatment in patients with obsessive compulsive disorder. *Indian Journal of Psychiatry, 62*(6), 684.

Neukirch, N., Reid, S., & Shires, A. (2019). Yoga for PTSD and the role of interoceptive awareness: A preliminary mixed-methods case series study. *European Journal of Trauma & Dissociation, 3*(1), 7–15.

Phillips, K. A., Coles, M. E., Menard, W., Yen, S., Fay, C., & Weisberg, R. B. (2005). Suicidal ideation and suicide attempts in body dysmorphic disorder. *Journal of Clinical Psychiatry, 66*(6), 717–725.

Rizzuto, L., Hay, P., Noetel, M., & Touyz, S. (2021). Yoga as adjunctive therapy in the treatment of people with anorexia nervosa: A Delphi study. *Journal of Eating Disorders, 9*(1), 1–12.

Saeed, S. A., Cunningham, K., & Bloch, R. M. (2019). Depression and anxiety disorders: Benefits of exercise, yoga, and meditation. *American Family Physician, 99*(10), 620–627.

Veale, D., Gledhill, L. J., Christodoulou, P., & Hodsoll, J. (2016). Body dysmorphic disorder in different settings: A systematic review and estimated weighted prevalence. *Body Image, 18*, 168–186.

Chapter 1

Yoga, Chanting and Eye Movement Desensitisation and Reprocessing for BDD from a Lived Experience Perspective

─────

ANNA WARHURST

Eyes open. I look from left to right. Still the same room, the same furniture sitting quietly around me. I treasure those first few moments after I wake up in the mornings. The rumination hasn't quite kicked in yet. I can almost sense that blissful peace Eckhart Tolle speaks about, that present awareness that pervades and fills the space around us.

My eyes cast down to my arm. BAM! The tingling starts, my heart begins to jump erratically, my breath becomes shallow. My eyes tremor and reverberate, with the image of my arm projecting back into my eyes, my brain; my skull begins to ache. It can't quite compute. It doesn't want to compute. There are no words, just a deep pervasive feeling of wrongness, which shudders through the rest of my body. The back of my neck tightens. My tongue wanders desperately, yet there are no words, just wordless confusion.

This is how I start most days, a pattern which continues throughout the day, and into the evening, over and over again. It is as though a wave washes over me, drowning me, robbing me of my ability to speak and voice this experience. I am numbed, pulled down into the trenches of my mind. I am lost.

On the surface, I get up, move around. My eyes cast around, looking, grasping for something to focus on in the outside world. I wonder what needs to be done, to keep myself moving. I brush my teeth, get myself breakfast, try to focus my energy on any external stimuli that might grab my attention: the shine of the familiar door handle, the roughness of the carpet, the light coming through the window. Underneath, all the while, this feeling festers, an inexplicable feeling of wrongness with myself, weighing down every movement I make, every second, as time ticks on.

Typical approaches to body dysmorphic disorder (BDD) measure the diagnosis by the amount of time spent preoccupied and distressed with the defect. 'One hour, three hours, six hours?' they ask. I turn to my mind for a calculation. It laughs back, *You're with this the whole time my friend*. I am filled with a sense of being deeply misunderstood, like my experience needs to be put into a neat black and white box to become real. It refuses to do so.

'When the thoughts come', they say, 'just think how you might think about the situation differently. What is the evidence to suggest your arm is not, indeed, the ugliest thing in the world? Just think about it and write down your thoughts.' They smile at me encouragingly, pleased with their suggestion. I turn to my arm and to the feeling, the wordlessness, the reverberations in my eyes. 'Yeah', I say, 'I'll give it a go.'

I turn on my laptop. It is time to attend another Zoom meeting. My reflection beams back at me, my eyes widen, stinging with disgust. *Just smile, what can you do? You are disgusting, and there's nothing you can do about it. Just ignore it, smile, and off we go. That big nose, big cheeks...you look like a man...and your teeth! Don't let them see your ears, at least cover them up.*

The meeting goes on. People's faces stare blankly back at me as I attempt to formulate words into sentences and paragraphs, hoping they can't hear the shake in my voice, the ugliness that leaks out from my every motion, every sound I make. All the while my lower back pulsates, my stomach tightens. At every opportunity my eye steals a look at my fleshy body below, the reflection of myself in the corner of the screen, like a drug I just can't resist, permeating every cell in milliseconds, rushing through me and all around me. It becomes a game. If I can just picture myself through their eyes, to the best of my ability, I am safe, I am ready for whatever the world throws at me. Just a quick glance will do it, but then I become hungry, I need more certainty, endlessly searching for a clearer picture of what I look like to them. The certainty never comes.

I shut the laptop, exhausted. I peel myself towards the next task. I must write down meeting actions, but what was even said? I don't know, I don't care. The feeling festers. What does it want? What am I even feeling? Is it sadness? Self-pity? Shame? Numbness? It's hard to tell.

'Just reframe your thinking' I hear the therapist's words ring in my ears. *How do I do that when I don't know what I'm thinking?* I wonder to myself.

My go-to in these moments is a mindful movement and chanting meditation. I go to the Kundalini Lounge website (Kundalini is a rhythmic form of yoga, from the lineage of the Sikh tradition), scouring through the content for my favourite video entitled 'How to become enchantingly beautiful'. The name of the video makes me chuckle. Anyone would think I was incredibly vain watching this. If they only knew...

The video starts with a gentle cat-cow movement to the sound of a soft Kundalini chant. Immediately, I feel my inner child stir up and pay attention. I've always loved music, especially gentle soothing rhythms. I'm transported back to long car journeys as a child, sitting in the back, gazing out of the window, mentally counting the passing cars to soothe me (early signs of obsessive compulsive disorder, they would say). I'd watch the raindrops trickle down the window, effortlessly making beautiful patterns and shapes. They would stare back at me, like strange ethereal faces, taking me to another world.

I begin chanting *Sat Nam*, the way we always start a Kundalini practice. Suddenly, I become aware of myself as a vocal, resonant being. I've got good at this. My mind quietens, and immediately the hopeless feeling that lingers around me, unspoken and unheard, begins to take a separate form. There is space between me and 'It'. I see it, I feel it: the space created around the inner pain. *Saaaat Naaaaam.* My mental attention skips from thing to thing, dancing from different pieces of sensory data, and at once I see my mind's movement, like a line graph swerving and scribbling its way up and down; I feel its movement through time and once again I find some peace. The gentle hum continues on, consistently and reliably in the background, cradling my mind, reminding me that I am here, connected to the outer world. Alive, whether I like it or not.

Experiences like this did not come immediately. They emerged over time. My meditation practice has become a necessary antidote to my daily experience, an intervention that provides me the space with which to rebalance my sensory experience back to a state of clarity: to slow down, allowing me to see the movement through space and time that makes up my experience. Rather than juttering through time and space like a pinball machine, my eyes can move smoothly, elegantly, from moment to moment. For me, this practice has become essential to my life.

Like the BDD itself, the degree to which this medicine soothes and supports me differs each day and exists on a spectrum. Sometimes, it is like sinking into a warm bath, easy and comforting. Other times, it is torturous, strained. I am resistant and it takes time. Either way, it has become a vital ingredient for me to exist in my body and mind each day. Without it, I am sucked into a warped and distorted world, one in which every movement is accompanied by a reverberating feeling-form-pattern that pulls me towards obsessional self-checking behaviours, and will not leave me alone.

After I practise, my inner world is filled with a sense of okayness, just like those few seconds after I wake up. My senses are heightened, but with clarity. I am alert to the sounds around me and to the sensations on my skin, but my relationship to them is one of companionship, solidarity and acceptance rather than rejection and shame.

It is very difficult to describe the wordless relationships we have with our bodies and the sensations within them. To even consider that we have a relationship to these senses of ours can seem very odd. Having a diagnosis of BDD forces you to enquire into these subtle relationships and interplays of feeling inside yourself. Because to not pay attention is not an option: it can lead to severe distress, and even suicide. Having this difficult experience of BDD invites us to come out of the cognitive stratosphere of words and things, and out of the mental gymnastics we typically partake in, to a world of pure raw emotion. Through a kind of internal gesturing, we can inhabit that pre-verbal space that calls us and is at once scary and very peaceful. It is here, I believe, we can find peace.

For me, what is afforded by Kundalini yoga practices is a way to enter into this pre-verbal space. The practice is a sort of moving walkway that propels you when you get stuck in an obsessional distortion and cannot see clearly. The profundity of the experience exists on a spectrum, yet is always there to a lesser or greater extent. Sometimes I am moved to tears by the release it offers me, as I surrender and let go of the need to control my perceived image, allowing a veil of peace to settle around me. At other times, I come away feeling energised, mobilised and awake, with a crutch of support that wasn't there before. Either way, I am always humbled by the consistent feeling of connectedness to something greater than myself. This feeling pierces through the adrenalised addiction to body-checking and offers me a hand of reassurance, an inner smile. What I find even more remarkable is that this reassuring hand, smile and knowing eye feel so familiar, and reset my ability to remember and reach for my past memories and experiences in rich, textural detail. In my experience, this can be one of the most upsetting and distressing aspects of BDD: the inability to recall one's own stories, and share in the collective memory of one's past; the inability to remember who one is and experience one's connection with the world. I am always so grateful for the element of reintegration the practice of yoga brings.

Eye Movement Desensitisation and Reprocessing for BDD: A Personal Account

A few months after writing the initial draft of this chapter, I was fortunate enough to work with an Eye Movement Desensitisation and Reprocessing (EMDR) practitioner specifically to treat my BDD. I had heard about the recent successes of EMDR for treating BDD and trauma, and felt compelled to give it a go. What unfolded was a journey of self-discovery I could never have imagined. It was a process I could not have embarked on without the support of a fellow expert-by-lived-experience and professional EMDR practitioner and facilitator. For me, EMDR has tackled the way emotions and memory were held within my body as physical pain, which had come about through internalised self-hatred. The bilateral stimulation technique (BLS), which Beverley Hutton describes in more detail in Chapter 12, opened up pathways I believe I could not have accessed myself.

EMDR is a therapeutic method which allows you to investigate your moment-to-moment experience while in a dreamlike state. In my case, it involves holding buzzers in each hand which vibrate intermittently to mimic and help stimulate the natural rhythm of REM sleep, which is appropriate for processing memories. Although the person being led through EMDR is conscious throughout, they are invited to move through and verbalise their experiences as they arise within them, starting with a target image or memory which triggers a strong emotion. Rather than thinking consciously about what the memory means to them and recounting any associated stories, it's as though a deeper, more intuitive intelligence takes over. This innate intelligence seems to draw links between different experiences in one's life which reveal what needs to be seen for healing and understanding to take place.

When I started EMDR sessions I had hit rock bottom. I had tried every method out there to manage and treat my BDD, with little success. The most fruitful treatments, as described in the first part of this chapter, were meditation practices, particularly chanting, which allowed me to connect with a deeper part of myself. From this deeper part of myself, I could view the troubling compulsions and experiences of self-consciousness at a distance – at least, enough to find some peace and quiet – and to use this as a launch pad from which to approach my life.

EMDR enabled me to turn on the floodlights, to see further and deeper within. Through BLS, and the encouragement of a professional EMDR therapist, I have been able to confront the thoughts and experiences within me that I alone refused to see and could not access. Like sitting on a train watching my life play out before me, I have been able to view the experiences I had as a child from the perspective of a compassionate observer, verbalising experiences which seemed too terrifying to utter at the time.

What has been most fascinating within this process is the way in which my pain symptoms have subsided over the course of the sessions. With a renewed sense of self awareness, to 'know thyself' as the ancient Greek maxim goes, I am more able to identify pain as an unmet emotional need, as opposed to a symptom of some physical ailment. More often than not, the physical pain is my inner child, feeling unheard and unseen, gripping on to some coping mechanism I required at the time to survive; and, in thus doing, blocking my ability to see and address my emotional needs. I am now able to watch this process play out, rather than having it stuck inside me as a painful feeling from which there is seemingly no cause and no way out.

I feel so honoured to have been given the experience of working with an EMDR practitioner to untangle the inner emotional terrain that has caused me so much trouble over the years: to understand it, piece it back together, and recognise that I am worthy and able to heal. I have developed a newfound respect for our inner natural intelligence, and increasing trust in allowing it to take over, knowing that it knows what needs to be done for healing to take place. While the journey has been scary at times, the layers of the onion continue to peel off, and I'm increasingly experiencing life with more and more presence. I am feeling grateful, interested and engaged with life, without the torturous BDD compulsions wreaking havoc in my daily experience. My memory and cognition are returning, and the felt sense of who I am and always have been has begun to flow back into me.

I believe interventions such as these, which allow us to tap into the unconscious mind, should be made available for experiences such as BDD which have underlying developmental and complex trauma at their core. I believe that we need to start recognising the experiences of BDD as symptomatic of trauma, so we can help people to access the holistic and trauma-informed approaches they need. In my case, it was only when I was granted the ability to access the entirety of my experience that I was able to begin the healing journey.

It is vital that those who need and want access to trauma-informed and embodied treatments are able to do so, so they can start living the life they yearn for and deserve. I hope my contribution to this book highlights the potential these methods can have to drastically change a person's experience. I also hope I have given an insight into the existential form BDD takes. With the hopelessness and high suicidality and suicide rate, it really is a matter of life or death. I hope this will be heard by both those who commission and those with the power and resources to help the multitudes of people experiencing BDD out there who need support and also have the innate potential to recover.

Chapter 2

The Neglected Trauma of Neglect

Considering Emotional Developmental Trauma in BDD

———

ARIE WINOGRAD

Body dysmorphic disorder (BDD) evolves from the intersection of multiple aetiologies including neurobiology, trauma, years of repetitive behaviours and aspects of the family system. Over the many years of working as a psychotherapist treating hundreds of clients with BDD, I have observed that one of the common denominators is that the family system typically plays a pivotal part. More overt causations of each individual's symptoms may differ: for instance, one person may have experienced systemic bullying in school whereas another may never have been bullied. Regardless, many years of clinical practice have taught me that the family system is a necessary focal point in the treatment of BDD. In this chapter we will explore how emotional developmental trauma, i.e. what *didn't* happen in childhood, can impact upon a person's felt sense of self and emotional regulation in the context of BDD.

Community has always been an essential element in the evolution of human beings: it has been our ability to work together and to share ideas and information which has increased our likelihood of survival. We can speculate that the emotion of loneliness, and the anxiety and depression that can occur with loneliness, evolved as a warning signal to seek out other humans since being physically alone would have decreased our chances of survival. Fast forward many millenniums and humans still experience loneliness, despite reduced overt danger of being physically alone. An attuned, supportive community provides the experience of physical safety along with emotional safety, and the family is our first group of people: our first community. In our families we learn how to navigate communal social interactions, as well as how to relate to others.

These very formative relational experiences become the template for how we learn to manoeuvre within the complexities of interpersonal relationships.

I have always said that one cannot consider BDD without considering interpersonal, and particularly intimate, relationships. Challenges with intimate relationships are a feature of BDD and one that cannot be ignored (Natalie Stechler explores the subject of intimate relationships in more detail in the next chapter). I am sure most clinicians who have treated BDD would agree that the discernible body image symptoms themselves interfere with an individual achieving nourishing intimacy. If a person believes they are too unattractive to be viewed by others, they will avoid or minimise human interactions. Many people with BDD spend hours a day performing compulsive behaviours in an attempt to ready themselves for contact with others; these rituals are undertaken in an attempt to minimise the emotional agony from possible rejection. Furthermore, if a person is having an intense relationship with a body part, this leaves much less space to have relationships with people.

Shame as a Foundation of BDD

Alongside the aspect of social interactions, the emotion of shame implicitly exists within the foundation of BDD (e.g. Veale, 2014). Shame is experienced as a deep sense that something is inherently wrong with oneself. Regulated shame is part of normal human development and felt by all of us to some degree within our lives. However, the person with BDD experiences shame, particularly unregulated or 'un-repaired' shame, as part of their developmental history, which leads them to believe their entire identity is bad and/or defective, or that by existing they must be a burden to humanity. In BDD, this shame is experienced through an aesthetic area or areas of the physical being the person perceives as defective. Somewhere along their life timeline they began to focus on this bodily feature; perhaps they were teased about it by peers or maybe their family of origin emphasised outward physical appearance. Or perhaps the individual does not know why they woke up one day intensively focused on a particular aspect of their appearance. Regardless, shame has become intrinsically associated with the physical appearance feature.

Although one experiences shame from within, shame is a highly socially based emotion as well as a visual emotion (e.g. Schore, 2015). An infant does not leave the womb experiencing shame. Rather, shame develops within the context of interpersonal relationships. The very first contact a newborn has with its mother and/or father, who are typically the primary caregivers, is where the human inter-relational mirroring experience begins. Emotional mirroring is a process by which a primary caregiver is emotionally attuned to the needs of an infant and, in turn, mirrors back to the infant a similar experience via facial expressions, voice intonation and touch. This is an imperfect process by which emotional misattunement inevitably occurs since no one person can absolutely and continuously mirror back the experience of another person. In secure attachments, these misattunements allow the 'rupture and repair' cycle to happen; these cycles are part of normal, healthy human development. However, if the ruptures are continually not repaired – if the caregiver continually misattunes with the infant without the repair of a loving gaze, a tender word, a hug etc. – the infant does not have a secure emotional base or sense of self from which to go out and explore the world.

An emotionally mature parent will be able to identify when a misattunement with their infant has occurred, then promptly reattune to their infant. It is during this process that a child grasps how to regulate their emotions, learning very early in life that emotions are not good or bad, right or wrong, but rather a natural human experience. The antecedents of entrenched shame are traumatic interpersonal experiences, especially those which occur in infancy or childhood. These traumas can be as overt as a child who is verbally, emotionally or physically abused or neglected by a parent or parents. However, shame deriving from trauma may originate not only from what happened but from what *did not* happen. Although some individuals with BDD have endured tangible traumas such as childhood physical or sexual abuse, many report they have not experienced trauma; often they report they had a good childhood and came from a 'good family' as they might describe it. Some individuals with BDD are mindful that they came from emotionally detrimental family systems but report that they are unable to identify any specific traumas during their childhood.

The Centrality of Emotional Developmental Trauma

In my experience, when I ask prospective clients during their initial consultation if they have experienced trauma, they rarely share any significant events during their lifetime which they would consider traumatic.

If shame is the foundational emotion sustaining the BDD experience, how does shame exist if there are no obvious interpersonal traumatic experiences from which the shame derived? *Emotional developmental trauma* is often the relational experience of what *did not* occur during a child's development. It is imperative that infants receive food, water and shelter to survive, otherwise they will perish. However, without sufficient nurture, an infant can survive physically but likely will be unable to thrive. Nurture entails the primary caregiver providing safety, attuned physical touch, comfort and information about the world, and also necessitates emotional attunement, emotional mirroring and emotional validation.

If a child is not provided with sufficient nurture, how could or would they know that something is lacking, or completely missing, in the formative years of their life? If emotional nurture is not provided to a child, they will not have a cognitive concept of an essential ingredient in their existence as lacking. Although an individual may not have intellectual insight that something indispensable is missing from their life, on an experiential level they can sense that something does not feel complete. Since what did *not* happen to an individual can be such a vague and ambiguous concept, the sad irony is that emotional developmental trauma is often itself neglected in the process of therapy. I have yet to experience a client entering treatment exclaiming that they have come to address what did not happen in their childhood. At the beginning of my career as a psychotherapist, I too overlooked many clients' emotional developmental trauma because I was overly focused on their distress from the overt body image symptoms.

In my experience, the most prevalent trauma experienced by individuals with BDD is emotional developmental trauma. In fact, I would assert that the majority of individuals with BDD have experienced some degree of childhood emotional developmental trauma, existing on a continuum from having had only partial emotional nurture needs provided by a primary caregiver, to the complete absence of any emotional mirroring, emotional validation or emotional attunement.

Often individuals minimise emotional developmental trauma, comparing it to the anguish of objectively conspicuous events such as physical or verbal abuse, which they believe are, and may describe as, 'real traumas'. The experience of being raised in a family system wherein some parents/caregivers and siblings are physically available yet simultaneously emotionally misattuned creates a profoundly lonely reality for a child. The child knows they are not actually alone, yet their experience is that of being disconnected from the other members of their family system who live under the same roof. The contrast between being with people while concurrently feeling emotionally abandoned leaves the child with an empty, void and incohesive internal experience. Many of my clients have described this feeling as if they are floating into the ether with nothing to tether themselves to.

Children depend on their parents for basic survival and will do anything to remain attached to them; this includes idealising the primary caregiver as all-powerful and who can do no wrong. Because the child experiences the primary caregiver as omnipotent, a paucity of emotional nurture is often processed internally as an inherent defect within themselves. The symptoms of BDD, then, become a tangible solution for the intangible experience of feeling intrinsically inferior and desperately alone.

BDD is, in itself, an extremely lonely experience. Besides the relentless negative intrusive thoughts about the aesthetic bodily feature deemed defective, the desolation endured can be equally if not more harrowing. There are numerous reasons why individuals with BDD usually refrain from speaking about their perceived aesthetic imperfections, and shame is absolutely embedded within this lack of self-disclosure. The physical feature of focus has become the epicentre of shame: in essence, shame concretised. To speak about or to draw further attention to this body area is experienced as exposing to another person their deepest feelings of being inherently defective, 'bad', 'detestable' and many similar sentiments besides.

To the person with BDD, there also exists the shame of feeling misunderstood or invalidated if something about their fraught relationship with a perceived defect is shared. To be told something like 'It looks fine, just stop worrying about it' is extremely invalidating: if they could stop the negative intrusive thoughts they would have already done so. Furthermore, the body area they are preoccupied with has become the barometer of their self-worth and identity, so invalidation surrounding this is typically experienced and internalised as a rejection. Even worse, to share the deeply personal experience of BDD and then to be proclaimed as vain is not only very shame inducing, but also sends the message to the person that no one truly understands what they are going through and, yet again, that they are alone.

The Relational Paradox of BDD

The paradox of BDD is that the person yearns to relate to, connect with and attach to people. However, the fear of possibly being rejected by others is so doused with shame that the option to avoid people is very tempting. BDD thrives when the person is isolated because there is no emotional mirroring or information from outside interpersonal interactions which can challenge the intransigent BDD message: *I will probably be rejected because of my appearance, and this will be the evidence solidifying my internal experience that there is something truly defective about me. And this confirms that I am not lovable.* Thus, interacting with others feels very risky for the person experiencing BDD because a rejection, or perceived rejection, activates such a dysphoric experience that to be by oneself by contrast may, at least temporarily, feel like the preferred option.

The paradox of BDD is such that the more the person focuses on the body part as a solution, the more they become disconnected from people. Equally, the more they become disengaged with people, the more they focus on the physical feature. The resulting struggles in human interactions will inevitably decrease the possibility of the person getting their basic human nurture needs met, especially those of emotional nurture.

In my experience, BDD can essentially recreate an individual's childhood of emotional malnutrition wherein a scarcity of human emotional mirroring, emotional attunement and emotional validation resulted in a disconnected, empty and deeply lonely inner experience. This BDD re-enactment of childhood emotional developmental trauma further fortifies the individual's already deeply ingrained idea that they will always be alone. Ironically, the person often ends up gazing into an actual mirror or similar reflective surface in an attempt to figure out what is so wrong with them. Unfortunately, the reflection from a physical mirror cannot provide what was never instilled in the first place; the emotional recognition that one is unconditionally lovable and the corresponding integrated sense of self that evolves when a child receives sufficient emotional nurture in their formative years.

When I speak with a client regarding the origins of what did or did not happen within their family system during their childhood, I emphasise that my motive is not to blame nor to condemn their parents or carers. However, I explain that it is important to explore their experience within the context of their family system. To blame would insinuate that a parent knowingly withheld nurture. If a parent had received adequate nurture from their own parents, they would have possessed the built-in capacity to provide emotional mirroring, affection, attunement and all the other necessary ingredients to create a secure attachment with their child. A parent who was raised in a family system with a paucity of nurture cannot instinctively create what they themselves never experienced, thus emotional developmental trauma is intrinsically *transgenerational*: trauma which is passed on from generation to generation, unless it is resolved.

The Early Parental Experience and BDD

A motif I have observed is that the majority of my clients who are experiencing BDD have parents who existed on opposite ends of the emotional spectrum: one parent was typically emotionally disconnected, disengaged or under-involved while the other parent was emotionally overwhelming, erratic or enmeshed with their child. Although this emotional pairing may work (on the surface) for a couple, it can create a poor developmental prognosis for the child or children who are born into an environment in which feelings exist on the extreme ends of the emotional continuum. For the child raised by this parental profile, it can be the case that if they turn to the emotionally disengaged parent for mirroring, there will not be adequate emotional reflection. When they turn to the emotionally dysregulated parent, on the other hand, they see a reflection of emotional disarray which is antithetical to healthy, good enough emotional mirroring. If the parent is emotionally over-engaged, the child does not learn how to regulate their own emotions. In any of these scenarios, a child's emotional development may be hindered, leaving them vulnerable to attempting to solve emotions via intellect or by seeking external resolution.

Indeed, the person experiencing BDD is seeking external resolution and attempting to regulate their emotions, as well as resolve trauma, by means of fixing or 'figuring out' an aesthetic bodily feature. BDD, in fact, tends to manifest as highly all-or-nothing, rigidly held beliefs about the body that become intrinsically linked to a person's self-value and identity. This differs from someone experiencing mild body dissatisfaction. An individual with body dissatisfaction does not like aspects of certain physical features; however, the epicentre of their identity does not evolve around the body part.

A healthy integrated identity develops within the context of adequate emotional nurture, appropriate parental boundaries, the opportunity to think and feel for oneself, and unconditional love. The formation of an integrated identity cannot develop with conditional love because a child is always performing for important, even essential, others rather than simply being who they truly are. Conditional love and the subsequent judgment create an internal experience of shame, and this pervasive shame directly interferes with identity formation (e.g. Schimmenti, 2012). Since shame is the internal experience that one must be inexplicably defective, bad, disgusting, a burden or irrelevant, the response to this can be to go towards external entities in an attempt to mitigate feeling inherently defective. If a child learns that love is conditional, their identity evolves within the context of the parent or parents' values, and this is antithetical to the development of one's own identity. A child who is raised with good enough emotional nurture is able to develop an internal sense of agency: the inner experience that one can shape one's own life.

Identity Formation in BDD

Shame as a social emotion occurs within the context of other people. When shame originates within the context of a parent—child relationship, the experience of being powerless (and thus inherently inferior) becomes the template of a child's identity. When shame erodes the formation of an integrated sense of self, grasping onto external experiences of objects can become the basis of identity. The experience of those who struggle with BDD is such that their identity forms around an external factor – a body part – while an inner sense of self does not evolve or is very fragile.

One of the many tragedies of emotional developmental trauma is that the formation of an individual's identity is disrupted. The invisible trauma of feeling incomplete, empty or disconnected is deeply intangible; when a child is unable to resource from within to feel whole, they look externally to fill the void. This is when and where symptoms develop and, in the case of BDD, symptoms evolve around a tangible aspect of an individual: their physical form. The body part becomes the conduit by which the person grapples with the internal experience of powerlessness and inferiority, while it is simultaneously held as a beacon of hope: *If only this body area looked somewhat normal, I would be okay*. The individual with BDD begins to engage in body-related checking compulsions in order to make sure that it *is* okay, which translates to *they will be* alright.

Compulsive behaviours are driven by hope that the body part will eventually be tolerable. However, hope never entirely arrives because there is no physical, body solution for an identity that never fully formed. As the individual struggling with BDD engages in more and more compulsions seeking hope, the unresolved shame that is at the core of BDD becomes displaced onto the perceived defect.

Almost every individual with untreated BDD will report that they become dysphoric when they view the perceived defect: this reinforces their belief that it is the defect which is responsible for their feelings of misery and unlovability. However, this may be a two-way street: as BDD evolves from emotional developmental trauma, the person never learned to regulate their emotions. When, therefore, they experience uncomfortable emotions – especially shame, guilt and loneliness – the experience is automatically attributed to the aesthetic feature deemed defective. If the infrastructure of an identity emerges from shame, external approbation and deficits in emotional regulation, the need for hope becomes paramount to one's existence. This is an extremely fragile foundation. The fragility and underdevelopment of identity in people experiencing BDD leaves them highly susceptible to interpersonal struggles beyond the overt body-related symptoms.

'Inside Out' and 'Outside In' Therapeutic Work

BDD derives from both internal and external factors, and all of these factors require emotional resolution. 'Inside out' therapeutic work entails processing emotions, especially shame and guilt, within the context of the therapeutic mirroring experience. This is an emotionally corrective process wherein the therapist provides an emotionally mirrored and attuned experience. 'Outside in' therapeutic work involves BDD-specific therapy that inevitably activates uncomfortable emotions – most frequently shame – which can then also be processed within the therapeutic mirroring environment. Since shame comes into fruition within the context of conditional love, judgment and emotional developmental trauma, the dissolving of shame must occur within the space of unconditional regard and good enough emotional mirroring. Since shame is at the emotional foundation of BDD, as well as the malefactor interrupting identity formation, without the mitigation of toxic shame a healthy identity cannot evolve and BDD will continue to thrive.

It is the longer-term therapeutic work of identity development that ultimately undermines the negative body image symptoms, hence the emphasis on shame resolution throughout the recovery process. The journey of individuating and integrating one's identity cannot, however, exist only within the confines of the therapy session. Identity integration involves going into uncomfortable emotions, including shame, while not seeking out a behaviour which temporarily mitigates the discomfort.

The process of addressing disconnected and dysregulated emotions from the inside out and outside in activates opportunities for the person to begin to internalise how to regulate their emotions from within rather than attempting to do so via a physical feature. Learning how to regulate emotions internally is significant in identity formation – a process which is stunted by emotional developmental trauma. As the person gradually begins to regulate their emotions from within, there becomes less need to regulate these emotions through a body part and through compulsive behaviours like mirror checking. Enduring uncomfortable emotions while having support during the process lays a solid foundation for a burgeoning identity: the opposite of an identity formulated around shame.

Navigating Family Systems

This chapter would not be complete without highlighting what a delicate process it is to navigate family systems where BDD is present. Whether or not the parents/caregivers need to be included in therapy is dependent upon the extenuating circumstances of the level of struggle in each particular family system. For mild or moderate BDD, there is usually less emotional developmental trauma, thus less interruption in identity formation. These are the cases where the person has likely already physically individuated from their family system; thus treatment may not necessitate involving the family directly. In severe and entrenched BDD, the recovery process may need to engage the family system to support positive outcomes.

If a parent or caregiver of someone with BDD is reading this, I want to commend them for taking the time to learn about BDD and how it can so significantly torment their child or loved one. Parents and carers almost always want the best for their children and do not wish to see their child suffer. Education about BDD is an appropriate first step. My number one recommendation to parents is to enter their own therapy. Yes, as a caring parent it is very important to reach out and be very supportive of your child; however, this is often insufficient. I often wonder if my clients would recover more rapidly if their parents simultaneously attended their own individual therapy. Besides the fact that BDD derives from the family system, it would send an overt message to the person with BDD that *we, the family, need to change in some way*, rather than *you need to change in some way*. When I make the recommendation to include family members in therapy, I explain that if the family expend all their efforts on trying to 'fix' their child they will likely be unable to see their own blind spots. Aspects which may be keeping the BDD going may, therefore, remain.

For a client in recovery from BDD and undergoing the related process of individuation, the extent to how much they remain involved in their family of origin is a very personal decision which is ideally supported by the therapist. As a client begins to experience a decrease of overt BDD symptoms, and as this coincides with the acknowledgment and better understanding of any emotional developmental trauma they experienced, the person often begins to experience grief: the grief of how significantly their childhood trauma changed the course of their lives, and where, or who, they could have been if the trauma had been identified and addressed earlier. It can be an intensely painful experience to realise that nourishing aspects were missing in one's childhood. The person may yearn for what might still be possible, but also harbour resentment towards the caregivers who missed the mark in providing good enough emotional nurture needs. Every child yearns to receive unconditional love from a parent and to have their parent truly understand them, but for those who experienced emotional developmental trauma, unconditional love and a healthy emotional connection may have been inconsistent or non-existent. Intellectually, the person understands that it is unlikely they will ever receive this from their parent(s), but experientially they still covet the emotional nurture which every child deserves.

Recovery from Emotional Developmental Trauma and BDD

The process of recovery from emotional developmental trauma, and its resultant body dysmorphic symptoms, involves people and community. A person may not have had a choice of their first community – their family – but as an adult they can embrace the company of people who fulfil their emotional needs. Just as BDD recovery involves physically and financially separating from the family system, becoming involved with a community is a behavioural facet of treatment. For individuals who have been isolated due to the severity of their symptoms, joining a community tends to be a longer-term goal in therapy and occurs once overt symptoms have been minimised. However, the gradual process of supporting the person to reach a point where they can begin to be involved with a community *they choose* is a greater goal of treatment. I explain to my clients that the purpose of everything we are doing is not just to reduce BDD symptoms, but to create the identity infrastructure that allows them to have a richer quality of life. The reduction of symptoms is part of this process, but to only focus on the obvious body-related symptoms misses the larger objective: recovery from emotional developmental trauma. This involves good enough mirroring experiences with people, including in the therapeutic space and in the community 'out there' in the world.

Emotional developmental trauma evolves from a group of people, thus recovery from emotional developmental trauma can only occur within the context of people. The confidential and safe space that exists within the confines of psychotherapy or similar is where this process can begin, and this creates the inter-relational framework for the person to take this corrective emotional experience and apply it to the outside world.

As the person becomes more involved with people, their BDD symptoms will likely exacerbate initially: an increase of human interaction means there are more people with whom they can compare themselves. Since the individual is already feeling inherently defective, they will likely conditionally judge themselves as inferior to others. More exposure to people also raises the possibility of rejection or perceived rejection. Body-related symptoms will usually manifest at this point because they protect the individual from the activation of archaic interpersonal trauma. BDD becomes more active when the individual increases interpersonal contact because it serves to protect against feelings of being inherently defective and inadequate. To make the choice to avoid people, however, will perpetually maintain the BDD experience. To choose to go towards people and communities will temporarily intensify body-related symptoms; however, it is also these relationships that will ultimately be integral to recovery from emotional developmental trauma, and therefore to recovery from BDD.

It is to be expected that as the world of people is entered, there will be many emotions that surface. These emotions need to be processed so the perceived aesthetic defect does not again become the conduit for these feelings. For those who have experienced emotional developmental trauma, going towards people and participating in communities can be frightening, arduous and emotionally activating. Getting to a point in recovery where one can begin to participate in interpersonal and communal relationships is a significant measurement of progress along the recovery journey. The reconstruction of one's identity from the solely external entities of appearance and performance to an internal experience of trusting oneself involves going into discomfort and tolerating this discomfort, while simultaneously having healthy-enough emotional mirroring experiences with people. The uncomfortable feelings that initially arise in these interpersonal interactions should not be avoided or replaced by body-related compulsions; rather, they can be embraced as an opportunity to learn how to regulate emotions internally rather than externally.

This stage of recovery is the antithesis of the conditions in which the emotional developmental trauma evolved. The individual is experiencing uncomfortable emotions, but rather than these feelings being ignored or invalidated, they are validated and mirrored back. This process, which may begin in the therapy office and then expands into the world, is a corrective experience which cultivates the formation of a true sense of self. The building and integration of an identity which is not founded in shame creates and supports an inner experience that is contrary to the empty, lost and lonely internal world that results from emotional developmental trauma. This inner experience consists of unconditional self-love, an understanding that one does not need to be perfect to be lovable, the ability to regulate emotions from within and the capacity to create healthy emotional mirroring to complement the internal emotional experience.

It is the integration of one's sense of self that supports an increase in the quality of interpersonal, communal and intimate relationships. When a person's identity is not saturated in shame, making oneself emotionally vulnerable presents less of a threat because there is no longer the trepidation associated with being exposed as defective. To make oneself more emotionally available creates a safe space for other people to do the same; it is within this space that emotional connection transpires.

Concluding Reflections

The antidote for emotional developmental trauma is authentic emotional connections with people. BDD cannot compete with genuine interdependent emotional relationships. The emotionally attuned and mirroring experience that occurs as two or more people are connecting overrides the BDD propaganda which states that one cannot be lovable unless they alter what is perceived as an aesthetic defect. The development of healthy emotional relationships gradually replaces the grieving caused by the realisation that parental emotional nurture may have been missing and might never occur. As shame acquiesces to trust, and as the fright of rejection is replaced by the safety of human connection, aesthetic bodily features serve much less of a purpose as a repository for unresolved emotional neglect.

For many, emotional developmental trauma is the intangible experience of what did not occur in childhood. Recovery from BDD is the opposite: reducing tangible symptoms while creating a foundation for what every person inherently deserves to experience – namely, unconditional love.

References

Schimmenti, A. (2012). Unveiling the hidden self: Developmental trauma and pathological shame. *Psychodynamic Practice, 18*(2), 195–211.

Schore, A. N. (2015). *Affect regulation and the origin of the self: The neurobiology of emotional development.* Routledge.

Veale, D. (2014). Shame in body dysmorphic disorder. In P. Gilbert & J. Miles (eds), *Body Shame* (pp. 281–296). Routledge.

Chapter 3

Adopting a Relational and Interpersonal Perspective when Working with Clients Experiencing BDD, Including Addressing Struggles Related to Physical Intimacy

NATALIE STECHLER

Humans do not exist in isolation. How we experience our bodies when interacting with others suggests that body image may be reciprocal in nature. This raises the question of what it is like to be in a relationship and experience being physically intimate when living with difficulties around one's body and appearance. This chapter highlights how relational and interpersonal dynamics lead to inevitable distress and vulnerability for the person living with body dysmorphic disorder (BDD) and their partners. It explores physical intimacy in the context of BDD, highlighting some key areas of importance around engaging in physical intimacy such as shame, projection, detachment, disembodiment and trauma.

BDD within a Relational and Interpersonal Context

Although part of the experience of BDD is personally subjective, due to each person's relatedness-to-the-world and inseparability from other people being unique and nuanced, relationships must be considered when understanding BDD. Cash, Theriault and Annis (2004) propose that body image disturbances must be viewed not only intrapersonally but also within an interpersonal context. As such, it is important for those living with BDD and clinicians working with BDD to look beyond how BDD is experienced from a purely intrapersonal perspective and consider the experience within a person's relationships.

Living with BDD affects many areas of a person's life, on an individual, systemic and interpersonal level. Despite there being a lack of research specifically addressing interpersonal struggles within BDD, it is clear that relationship difficulties form a central aspect (for example, Brohede et al., 2016; Didie et al., 2012; Phillips, 2009; Silver & Reavey, 2010). Social inhibition, non-assertiveness and sensitivity to rejection by others all appear to be contributing factors to BDD (Didie et al., 2012; Fang et al., 2011).

The person experiencing BDD can find it difficult to be around and trust others and to socialise, due to the preoccupation with their appearance and their feelings of unattractiveness. The fear of being perceived negatively by others can result in an inability or struggle to form relationships. Feelings of imprisonment and of being restricted in one's capacity to comfortably make relational connections are also commonplace for people experiencing BDD, specifically with concerns around family or friends and difficulties with intimate partners.

Typical relationship struggles for people experiencing BDD include: (1) a lack of time for partners due to ritualistic behaviours, including relationships interrupting ritualistic safety behaviours and coping strategies; (2) a partner's lack of understanding and patience; and (3) a feeling that partners would be better off without them. It can be a struggle for people with BDD to comprehend how others would want to be in a relationship with them, or could see them as attractive, given their intensely negative self-perceptions. The individual living with BDD can often feel as though their partner is yet to see the real version of themselves, which they believe is defective and flawed (Silver & Reavey, 2010). A fear of being rejected by a partner, or potential partner, can be central to the experience of BDD.

Aesthetic Objects and Objectification

When discussing relationships in the context of BDD, it is helpful to consider objectification theory: in particular, self-objectification wherein the self is processed as an aesthetic object. Individuals who self-objectify appear to view themselves as an aesthetic object and, therefore, that they are only perceived by others according to their physical appearance, rather than perceiving themselves holistically, including subjective, non-observable elements.

When individuals with BDD construct their sense of self in the mind, appearance is the primary focus (Veale, 2001). People experiencing BDD fear that the self is seen by others as only ugly and deformed. The value and focus they place on their external self amplifies this viewing of the self as an aesthetic object.

Individuals with BDD judge and compare themselves against an internalised, unrealistic ideal which is based purely on physical appearance. As such, through a process referred to as self-objectification (Fredrickson & Roberts, 1997), the self is processed as an aesthetic object, evoking body shame and appearance-related behaviours (Lambrou, Veale, & Wilson, 2011). Self-worth in relationships within the context of BDD, then, becomes dependent on appearance and how positively or negatively the appearance is perceived to be judged by others. Taking such a stance, the body becomes a 'thing' of inquiry to be evaluated, manipulated and controlled.

Shame in the Gaze of the Other

The gaze of another, including embodied experiences in relating to others, is significant in the context of BDD and relationships. Being around others exposes those who are preoccupied with their appearance to the so-perceived harsh gaze of others. The gaze of another can significantly impact upon how individuals view and engage with their body in relation to others.

Being seen or watched may underline a primary anxiety, eliciting feelings of being judged by others who could see the person experiencing BDD as ugly and unlovable (Lemma, 2009). Philosophical discourse suggests that shame is an aspect of being seen: 'shame is the incorporated gaze of the Other' (Fuchs, 2002, p. 228). Indirectly, the feeling of shame draws awareness of the Other's gaze (Fuchs, 2002). Philosopher Jean-Paul Sartre (1969) posits that we can have no absolute certainty or confirmation over our perception of the Other's gaze, as it is removed from our own visual perception. We are left only with our suspicions and the fear that other people will judge us and perceive us negatively. Fuchs (2002) suggests that it is through being looked at that shame around one's appearance and body is evoked.

According to Sartre (1969), the body is invisible until the presence of the gaze makes it visible. Under the gaze of the Other, our lived-body becomes a visible object which is subject to the Other's existence. Through the gaze of the Other, the lived body no longer exists in and of itself but, rather, as the body-for-others.

People often perceive and make sense of their physical appearance through observing the desired object, such as their partner. The gaze objectifies the lived body and can prevent a person from being in the present moment. The gaze can also restrict one's bodily-being and produce the feeling of being forced to 'put on' a self-performance, by playing a role or persona when in relationships. Sartre highlights that dislike of one's body can manifest in a wish to be 'invisible' and 'not to have a body anymore' (Sartre, 1969, p. 353). People experiencing BDD long to hide from view and will engage in behaviours such as staying indoors alone, and concealing or camouflaging in an attempt to make invisible the perceived defects to the gaze of the Other. Indeed, an aspect of BDD is the hiding of one's authentic self and body from one's partner in an attempt to conceal a true self that is felt to be flawed. As such, one's natural and spontaneous bodily existence is 'hijacked' under the gaze of the Other. Thus, the person is left experiencing the self as an object of attention (Fuchs, 2002).

Perception and Mentalisation

People with BDD can experience an intense sense of unworthiness within relationships, often questioning their worthiness around appearance rather than judging their worth in relation to their whole being. As people experiencing BDD view themselves as deformed, flawed and ugly it can be difficult for them to believe that their partners do not share these same beliefs. People with BDD often lack awareness that their partners have their own mind; that they might not see and judge them as they see and judge themselves. This inability to separate their view of themselves from their partner's view of them can leave a person with BDD confused and even questioning why their partners are with them. The perceived judging and evaluative gaze, thoughts and feelings can be seen as a projection of the person's own judgment onto their partners' gaze, thoughts and feelings. One cannot know what their partner *is* actually thinking, only what *they think* their partner must be thinking about their body and appearance.

As such, attending to how an individual with BDD approaches their partner's mind is important when exploring relationships in therapy, including gently challenging the belief that their partners must feel or think the same way. Mentalisation refers to one's capacity to attend to and make sense of the subjective mental states (thoughts and feelings) of oneself and others. This includes how one perceives and interprets the Other's intentional mental states. One can never be certain of what exists in the Other's mind. Therefore, when interacting with the Other, one creates beliefs about the Other's mental state, which can be shaped by one's own internal mental states and processes. The ability to mentalise involves the capability to separate one's own mental states from those of another. Supporting clients with mentalisation can therefore be a very important aspect of the therapeutic process with a person experiencing BDD.

Physical Intimacy

A particular area of difficulty to navigate within relationships when living with BDD is the interpersonal dynamic of being physically intimate in a relationship. Physical intimacy is a time and space within which the body is potentially exposed or seen. Perceptions of appearance and body can relate to the frequency and quality of sexual experiences, for example, with others (Cash et al., 2004). Sexual experiences with a partner place the person with BDD in a position wherein they are being seen and subjected to another's gaze. Sexual intimacy can, therefore, be imbued with a sense of being evaluated (Calogero & Thompson, 2009).

Physical intimacy in relationships forms a part of the interpersonal struggle for people experiencing BDD. There is often immense fear and difficulty around being naked, being touched and having intercourse. To varying degrees, a person with BDD can find touch and nakedness distressing, unsafe and suffocating; and, at times, they find themselves with no sex drive or ability to derive sexual pleasure (Brohede et al., 2016; Phillips, 2009; Silver & Reavey, 2010). Physical intimacy, and specifically intercourse, can become disembodied and non-relational; an act to be done (to), rather than experienced (with the Other). Physical intimacy can come across to the partner of someone with BDD as rigid and controlled. Detachment, disengagement or dissociation may be used to manage the shame and trauma triggered by being physically intimate.

Shame and Projection in the Partner's Gaze

Experiencing one's body in relation to one's partner's body typically evokes a high degree of shame for a person with BDD. A partner's gaze on the naked or partially naked body can feel deeply painful and shameful as the body is exposed and vulnerable to the partner's judgment. It is important to hold in mind that it is the person with BDD's own judgment that is being projected onto their partner's gaze, feelings and thoughts. This highlights the importance of attending to the notion of both shame and projection when working with, and conceptualising, BDD and relationships.

The shame of being seen can lead a person with BDD to hide and camouflage themselves with objects, lighting, clothing or make-up. They might find themselves attempting to control and manoeuvre their partner's gaze as a means of managing discomfort during physical intimacy. When finding themselves in situations where they can't realistically escape being naked or exposed (such as during showering or sex, for example) they may find other ways of creating protection and a sense of safety to conceal the perceived flawed body parts (and the associated shame). Again, the assumption typically exists that partners will see them in the same flawed light, rather than the person with BDD considering that their partner may have different perceptions and judgments to their own.

The discomfort a person with BDD experiences with their body, alongside feelings of shame, inadequacy and disgust, present as barriers to immersion in the sensory and pleasurable experience of physical intimacy. This typically includes the need to disengage from bodily senses to cope with the unbearable feelings of being connected with the body in the context of physical intimacy. It can be difficult for people experiencing BDD to find pleasure in the act of intimacy; rather, it can become a source of stress or a mundane chore to be finished as quickly as possible. Sex can feel like an ordeal: something that has to be done rather than experienced and enjoyed. It is almost as though the sex becomes non-relational, no longer something to be experienced with the Other. The experience of another's touch can evoke strong physiological responses of anxiety, disgust and nausea also.

The Unwelcome Other

BDD often seems to take on an identity of its own, almost as though there are three people in a relationship, one of whom is a critical observer. BDD is not experienced as a welcome Other but, rather, as a source of distress and struggle, including during physical intimacy. BDD tends to take the form of a relentless critical Other who takes one away from being bodily-present and in the moment, and towards a more cognitive realm in which one is monitoring and evaluating the appearance of the body. Rather than being immersed or thinking about their partner's sensual experience of physical intimacy, a third-person perspective is often therefore adopted.

Working with BDD and Relationship Difficulties

It is clear that BDD makes intimate relationships difficult, unbearable even. What can be done to help? Attention to interpersonal functioning is recommended when working with BDD. Psychological assessments and formulations would ideally include an individual's cognitions, emotions and behaviours in relation to interpersonal and relational experiences. This includes an exploration of how the fixation and preoccupation with one's appearance impacts on the relationship between the person with BDD and their partner. Psychological interventions could helpfully attend to specific experiences within relationships, such as physical intimacy, nakedness, showering, dressing in front of the Other and/or sexual intercourse. Possible areas for exploration include shame in being seen, pain and detachment during physical intimacy, and sense of self-worth in the relationship.

Working with Shame and Trauma

In BDD, the shame related to one's appearance, and the shame of being seen in relationships, highlight the importance of psychological interventions focused on addressing shame. One of the therapeutic goals, therefore, is to build the ability to self-soothe and reduce feelings of shame and trauma through moving towards compassion and empathy.

Brené Brown (2012), a leading shame researcher, highlights appearance and body image concerns as a key trigger for shame. Shame is an intense and painful emotion, leading to feelings of entrapment, powerlessness and disconnection. Seeing oneself as flawed, not good enough or a failure leads to a sense of unworthiness in relationships, including how one perceives how their partner views them. In working towards change, Brown encourages attention to understanding what triggers shame, the importance of speaking about shame and cultivating self-awareness of shame. The goal is to move towards a stance of empathy and compassion.

Compassion Focused Therapy could be considered when working with people with BDD to help them to build an ability to self-soothe and to reduce feelings of shame (Gilbert, 2011; Veale & Gilbert, 2014). The aim is to move away from the highly active threat system when relating with others (including during physical intimacy) towards a more compassionate self. This includes noticing and turning towards distress rather than dissociating or avoiding it altogether. Holding a sense of compassion involves acknowledging, understanding and empathising, and a 'not your fault' approach to distress and suffering.

In order to nurture self-compassion and alleviate trauma and shame related to the experience of being physically intimate, the following aspects would helpfully be addressed:

- Any critically negative self-appraisals such as *I am flawed, ugly, deformed, worthless.*

- Beliefs such as *My partner must see me the way I see myself.*

- The need to hide, conceal, camouflage and control oneself and the environment due to a sense of worthlessness, inferiority and shame in relationships.

- The physiological effects triggered by shame and trauma such as the fight, flight, freeze and/or fawn response.

As you will read about in more detail in Rosa Hernando Hontoria's chapter (Chapter 11), Compassion Focused Therapy (CFT) postulates that shame persists when an individual has an imbalance between the three emotion regulation systems which are used to manage emotions (threat, drive and soothing systems). The threat system gets activated when there is perceived threat such as the gaze of a partner or physical touch, and will respond to situations, imagery and emotions such as shame, fear of rejection, self-criticism and any perceived loss of control. The emotional response of fear and anxiety triggers a protective fight-or-flight response wherein a person might avoid physical intimacy, or dissociate or withdraw while being physically intimate.

The drive system in CFT is associated with motivation and the pursuit of goals and achievements. Although it is linked to positive emotions, it can also drive behaviours involved in trying to escape the threat-based emotional and physiological responses. Such a pursuit often reinforces or exacerbates the distress. While engaging in physical intimacy, people with BDD typically strive towards controlling and manoeuvring a partner's gaze through camouflaging or hiding the perceived flaws, as previously described.

The soothing system, on the other hand, is associated with calmness and safety. This system helps to cultivate an ability to self-soothe in order to regulate the threat system. During times of distress, such as being physically intimate, the soothing system can be undeveloped or limited. The consequence of the threat system (e.g. being seen) and drive system (e.g. the need to hide and conceal an aspect of the body to prevent the partner seeing the flawed self) being so powerful and imbalanced against the soothing system is that the shame, trauma and sense of worthlessness in relationships and physical intimacy is maintained and even amplified. At times of distress, such as physical intimacy, a non-existent or under-utilised soothing system can often exist. Therefore, skills such as attention and mindfulness training, compassionate imagery (imagining a safe place) and compassionate mind or self (considering how the compassionate aspect of the self would react or feel) are important skills to explore and practise with clients.

Challenging Self-Worth in Relationships

As discussed earlier in the chapter, it is highly typical for a person experiencing BDD to confine their sense of worthiness within intimate relationships to their physical appearance. It is difficult for people with BDD to perceive and appreciate the other aspects of themselves they bring to the relationship such as non-observable characteristics, personality traits etc. Therefore, therapy can helpfully include an exploration of other traits and characteristics a person brings within their connection with others. This includes supporting clients to redirect their attention from appearance-focused aspects to other possibilities. One may begin by supporting a client to create a list of non-appearance-related traits and gifts they possess and can offer out to others, for example a sense of humour, kindness, a capacity for empathy and so on. The hope is to challenge the belief that appearance is central to one's self-worth in a relationship and more generally, and to support the person to thicken the narrative of who they are – of their felt sense of self – beyond the appearance of the physical body and the shame attached to this.

Working with the Mind–Body Connection

As discussed, experiencing nakedness, shared touch, sensual proximity, sexual contact and a wide range of other activities (including sexual intercourse) can lead to high levels of anxiety, shame and trauma in people experiencing BDD. This is often managed through dissociation and detachment. As such, clinical practice with this client group can helpfully include interventions which focus on supporting and nurturing a felt sense of connection with the body. For example, practitioners could embed embodied and body-focused aspects into their clinical practice with this client group, perhaps including mindfulness-based practices, to help clients focus on their bodily sensations as a means of coming into the present moment in their body. Some recommended approaches include:

- Supporting your client to bring their attention to their breath, as explored in more detail in other chapters of this book (e.g. Chapter 8).

- Yoga, Tai Chi and other breath-led movement practices (as explored in Chapters 6, 7 and 8).

- Embodied therapeutic modalities such as sensorimotor psychotherapy or 'trauma centre trauma-sensitive yoga' (TCTSY) therapy.

- Engaging with the eight senses to redirect one's attention to non-appearance-related cognitions. This is important as cultivating emotional and physical connectedness with the present moment can reduce the negative self-talk, shame, detachment and dissociation. Engaging with sensory experiences helps to narrow one's focus, which can, in turn, support an embodied and connected experience with one's partner (see Chapter 5).

People experiencing BDD have often become more familiar with 'being in their head' than 'being in their body' due to the intense preoccupations and fixations on appearance and resultant safety behaviours. Therefore, embodied techniques typically take time, patience and practice. It can be helpful to try these techniques with your client first in non-BDD-specific situations which feel less vulnerable and exposing.

Working with Couples

When working with couples wherein one partner is living with BDD, practitioners can helpfully acknowledge physical intimacy as a possible area of difficulty, emotional pain and/or detachment. They can helpfully take a curious stance and ask open, exploratory questions as to whether there are any difficulties that exist within particular intersubjective spaces such as nakedness, showering, dressing in front of the Other and/or sexual intercourse. The acknowledgement of both parties' subjective experiences is important, in order to allow for a better understanding of what it is like for both people in the relationship to live with the experience of BDD.

Where comfortable for the client (and their partner) and where appropriate, the partner of the person with BDD may be invited to attend some (or part of some) of the client's therapeutic sessions: to share their experiences and collaboratively surface difficulties and find ways forwards. Validation of each of the persons' experiences is vital and fundamental, and this will likely go some way too in reducing feelings of shame.

It can also be helpful to think together how the partner of the person with BDD might helpfully respond/react and act during times of physical closeness and intimacy. In addition, it is important to provide the person with BDD with opportunities to hear their partner sharing a different perspective to their own on their appearance and struggles.

The Therapeutic Relationship

The exploration of intimacy can bring up a tremendous amount of shame for the person experiencing BDD. Translated into the therapeutic space, the therapist's gaze could predispose a client to similar feelings of shame around being seen. The client and therapist do not exist in isolation but, rather, their subjective sense of self is mutually experienced. One could argue that being in therapy is an intimate experience: while the client is not physically naked, their physical body exists in an enclosed space in relation to another. Furthermore, the client naturally exposes aspects of themselves (such as emotions, thoughts and beliefs) within this therapeutic space. As such, the experience of shame in being seen is an important area to explore within therapy of any modality when working with clients with BDD. Some useful questions for therapists to ask their clients might be:

- What is it like to sit in relation to a therapist who is looking at you?

- What are you doing to avoid or reduce this gaze? Examples include avoiding eye contact and carefully angling the body away from light sources in the room.

- Are you looking for ways to protect yourself when you feel you can no longer hide from the therapist's gaze? What ways do you protect yourself at such times?

- Does the gaze of the therapist make you feel as though your body is somehow subject to evaluation? What might soothe this feeling?

It can be helpful to explore any perceptions a client might have of their partner's or therapist's gaze and to challenge their thinking in open, gentle and compassionate ways.

Acceptance and Compassion

Regardless of any experience of BDD, relationships in general tend to be complex and at times can feel messy and challenging, whilst also hopefully offering joy and a source pleasure of course. It can be helpful to remind clients that there is no such thing as a perfect relationship and that intimacy within relationships can be emotionally and physically difficult to navigate for many people, and can ignite strong feelings of vulnerability. At the same time, this vulnerability allows for the possibility of connectedness with others.

Clients with BDD can be helpfully supported to offer themselves patience and compassion when navigating relationships and the intimacy and vulnerability they bring, which can be modelled by the therapist. It is important to remind clients that it is completely usual and normal to feel uncomfortable with intimacy at times for all human beings, regardless of a struggle with BDD. This is not to say, however, that the additional struggles BDD brings should not be validated and explored.

It can also be helpful to explore any internalised familial, cultural or societal messages about physical intimacy and sex that clients may have assimilated, such as that sex should 'always be fun' or that 'intimacy should always feel romantic'. 'Always', 'never', 'should' and 'must' ideas can be gently unpacked and challenged, including a curiosity about where such messages may have come from and whether or not they are serving and supporting the client's experience and journey.

Concluding Reflections

This chapter has highlighted the importance of attending to the relational and interpersonal experiences and consequences for someone living with BDD. It has explored the importance of conceptualising and working with BDD within an interpersonal context, as well as from an intrapersonal perspective. It has emphasised how a person's negative appraisal of self, and heightened appearance-related concerns, can enter the intersubjective space of physical intimacy in relationships in particular.

As we have explored, perceiving oneself and one's body through a purely objectified lens can cause intimacy to become a disembodied experience. Alongside this, having a strong sense of worthlessness and a feeling of not being good enough can leave a person questioning why their partners are with them in the first place. Psychological interventions can therefore helpfully focus on addressing shame, trauma and the person's sense of unworthiness in physically intimate relationships by supporting the cultivation of compassion, mentalisation, self-worth, the ability to self-soothe and growth in self-acceptance.

References

Brohede, S., Wijma, B., Wijma, K., & Blomberg, K. (2016). 'I will be at death's door and realize that I've wasted maybe half of my life on one body part': The experience of living with body dysmorphic disorder. *International Journal of Psychiatry in Clinical Practice, 20*(3), 191–198.

Brown, B. (2012). *Daring greatly: How the courage to be vulnerable transforms the way we live, love, parent, and lead.* Penguin.

Calogero, R. M., & Thompson, J. K. (2009). Potential implications of the objectification of women's bodies for women's sexual satisfaction. *Body Image, 6*(2), 145–148.

Cash, T. F., Theriault, J., & Annis, N. M. (2004). Body image in an interpersonal context: Adult attachment, fear of intimacy and social anxiety. *Journal of Social and Clinical Psychology, 23*(1), 89–103.

Didie, E. R., Loerke, E. H., Howes, S. E., & Phillips, K. A. (2012). Severity of inter-personal problems in individuals with body dysmorphic disorder. *Journal of Personality Disorders, 26*(3), 345–356.

Fang, A., Asnaani, A., Gutner, C., Cook, C., Wilhelm, S., & Hofmann, S. G. (2011). Rejection sensitivity mediates the relationship between social anxiety and body dysmorphic concerns. *Journal of Anxiety Disorders, 25*(7), 946–949.

Fredrickson, B. L., & Roberts, T. A. (1997). Objectification theory: Toward under-standing women's lived experiences and mental health risks. *Psychology of Women Quarterly, 21*(2), 173–206.

Fuchs, T. (2002). The phenomenology of shame, guilt and the body in body dysmor-phic disorder and depression. *Journal of Phenomenological Psychology, 33*(2), 223–243.

Gilbert, P. (2011). Shame in psychotherapy and the role of Compassion Focused Therapy. In R. L. Dearing & J. P. Tangney (eds), *Shame in the therapy hour* (pp. 325–354). American Psychological Association.

Lambrou, C., Veale, D., & Wilson, G. (2011). The role of aesthetic sensitivity in body dysmorphic disorder. *Journal of Abnormal Psychology, 120*(2), 443–431.

Lemma, A. (2009). Being seen or being watched? A psychoanalytic perspective on body dysmorphia. *The International Journal of Psychoanalysis, 90*(4), 753–771.

Phillips, K. A. (2009). *Understanding body dysmorphic disorder.* Oxford University Press.

Sartre, J. P. (1969). *Being and nothingness.* Philosophical Library.

Silver, J., & Reavey, P. (2010). 'He's a good-looking chap ain't he?': Narrative and visualisations of self in body dysmorphic disorder. *Social Science & Medicine, 70*(10), 1641–1647.

Veale, D. (2001). Cognitive-behavioural therapy for body dysmorphic disorder. *Advances in Psychiatric Treatment, 7*(2), 125–132.

Veale, D., & Gilbert, P. (2014). Body dysmorphic disorder: The functional and evo-lutionary context in phenomenology and a compassionate mind. *Journal of Obsessive-Compulsive and Related Disorders, 3,* 150–160.

Chapter 4

Obsession and Me

BDD, Hyper-Focus, Creativity and Healing

———

ALEX MUMMERY

I was not born with body dysmorphic disorder (BDD). Indeed, BDD most typically begins to emerge during early adolescence. However, I do believe I was born with an obsessive-compulsive profile, or what could be described as in-built tendency to fixate on things that most other people would not. This propensity to fixate, particularly on aesthetic detail, is the focus of this chapter, alongside how art and creativity have been supportive to my recovery from BDD.

When I was five years old, my mum remembers how I would stop to pick up each and every piece of litter I passed on the walk home from school, stuffing them all into my little pockets. If she tried to intervene, I would sharply resist, which was generally uncharacteristic of me. In the end, she reconciled herself to an hour-plus journey back along the three or four streets between school and home. When I was seven years old, on a day out at the park, I remember my parents telling me it was time to head home. This triggered within me an overwhelming urge to touch every piece of equipment before we left, which I imagine caused them both confusion and frustration.

When I was nine years old, while visiting the local travelling fairground, I remember my dad trying and failing to win a prize at the coconut shy. I don't think I had even particularly coveted the prize in question, but my mind had already latched on to the idea of receiving it, and I remember feeling an itchy and insistent feeling that led to a prolonged period of distress that felt unusual and embarrassing even to myself. At the age of 11, I would rewatch the same portion of the same movie each day on my return home from school. I might spend two months rewinding my favourite half-hour of *Back to the Future*, before perhaps eventually switching to three months of the last act of *Star Wars*. It was only when I reached the age of 13 that my fixations began to focus on my appearance.

Through researching BDD for my doctoral thesis, I have come to wonder if there are at least two somewhat distinct paths to developing BDD. There is a strong link between BDD and traumatic childhood experiences, particularly events that centred on someone's physical appearance, be it teasing and bullying at school, or an inherited sense from one's family that appearance is important for happiness and success, leading to an embedded sense that personal worth comes from being physically attractive. Unfortunately, a lot of these experiences inhibit us from feeling self-worth within other areas of our lives. So when our appearance doesn't meet the unattainable expectations we have set, it can become a fixation.

There is also some research evidence that BDD has a genetic component: among people experiencing BDD, there is a high frequency of extended family members who would also meet the criteria for a diagnosis. Environmental factors can of course be shared within families, and correlation does not always equal causation, but large studies of twins have also established a strong genetic link for BDD (pairs of identical twins show significantly higher rates of co-occurrence of BDD than non-identical pairs). Although environmental and genetic factors are likely to combine in differing ratios for people with BDD, I personally identify as being more in the 'born obsessive' camp. In other words, it would seem to me that my natural propensity to fixate laid the groundwork for BDD to develop during the period in which adolescents begin to take more notice of the way they look, and how their appearance differs to that of other people.

I do not mean to state that environmental causes were not involved in the development of my own personal BDD, just that they were perhaps involved to a lesser extent than for others. I do believe that BDD will always have some environmental catalyst, and I have often tried to trace back to mine. I have arrived at a few potential events. Firstly, I have a memory of quite innocently commenting on an aspect of my sister's appearance, which unfortunately upset her. This angered my dad, who in uncharacteristic form retaliated by pointing out the prominent teeth I had at the time (pre-orthodontics), something I was already highly sensitive about. I remember feeling an intense mix of emotions: shame from the impact of my careless words, fear from the jarring experience of a caregiver striking at my insecurities, and despair at the realisation that other people were quite aware of my physical imperfections.

Although a flashbulb memory of shame, my BDD symptoms still did not develop for many years after the incident with my dad. Interestingly, I think I can pinpoint the exact moment they did. I had a close friend at school with whom I shared too many characteristics. This caused friction, the kind that can spark from the points at which people's personalities rub against each other. Basically, we were too similar to one other, and the feeling of seeing ourselves reflected back in the other person was aggravating. I used to tease my friend about being overweight, much to my shame now, and this led him to develop his own insecurities, insecurities I would later learn would probably also be best described as BDD. After one too many comments about his size, my friend sought out an aspect of my appearance he could exploit for retaliation. One day, quite out of the blue, during an English lesson, he said to me:

'You know, you have a strange-shaped head.'

'I do?' I said, quite perplexed. 'What do you mean?'

'It's too tall and narrow,' he said and turned away from me.

I remember the exact moment clearly. Having a strange-shaped head had not crossed my mind before and so it immediately confused me. It also quickly began to play on my mind. Directly after the lesson, I headed to the bathroom to look in the mirror, to see if he was right. I looked carefully, examining different areas of my head in turn. Perhaps my cheekbones were quite narrow compared to some other people. Maybe the top of my head was a little taller than most people's. This gave me an uneasy, nauseous feeling, but I was able to put it out of mind and continue with my day at the time. But the seed that had been planted from this one small comment from my friend was about to grow roots that would bury deep into my psyche. I would not be able to put that uneasy feeling out of my mind so easily for much longer.

BDD crept in slowly. At first, I would find myself lingering by the mirror for a few extra seconds, slowly turning my head left and right to examine its contours. Then I would find myself getting stuck in the mirror for minutes at a time, sometimes using a second handheld mirror to examine myself from various angles. I remember distinctly trying to get an objective reading on my appearance. How did I look to other people?

What did they see? Why had my friend chosen to say that about me, of all the things he might have picked on me for? (I've asked him more recently and he has no recollection of the event, and he certainly didn't agree with the comments of his past self!) Before long, I was using the family digital camera to photograph and video myself for up to an hour at a time. I was chasing a feeling of equilibrium, and sometimes I would find it: if a picture pleased me, I would feel a wave of euphoria – 'At last, I like this image, this is what I look like!' I would put down the camera and rejoin my family in the living room. However, this calm would only last for a few minutes before the creeping feeling of unease would begin to reform in the pit of my stomach. I would feel that itchy feeling I had felt when I *needed* to pick up each piece of litter from the street as a child, or when I *had* to touch each piece of equipment at the playground before we left. I would quietly stand up, return to the bathroom, lock the door, and re-enter the nightmarish loop of capturing and checking my image, feeling almost sick with anxiety at each photo until one, for whatever unknown reason, would soothe me.

My obsessions did not stop with what I would now refer to as 'checking'. In one way or another, my BDD consumed every waking minute of my life. One of my most frequent behaviours was making comparisons to other people. Sitting in class, I would examine the head-shape of every peer, searching for someone whose head was similar to mine. At home, I would Google famous celebrities, desperate to find someone successful with a strange-shaped head. Of course, as anyone who has experienced BDD will attest to, this was an impossible task. To me, I stood alone. I was distinct and separated from all other human beings, like some visiting cone-headed alien. Gradually, this thought began to make me convinced that I would never be happy or fulfilled, that no other person would ever be able to look past the shape of my head and love me. I envied people whose physical flaws were to do with weight, or their facial features, as these could be changed with exercise or surgery. There was no way that I would ever be able to change the shape of my head, which I believed was my only way out of this misery.

In hindsight, I'm very lucky there is no way to change the shape of one's head (believe me, I looked into it!) because I probably would've tried it. But what I was able to do was to grow my hair long, and so began the next of my obsessive behaviours: disguising. With my hair a certain length, I could style it so it would make my head appear broader, which became a daily morning ritual of indeterminate length. Throughout the day, each unforeseen rainfall, each glance into a passing car window, each misread glance from another person would trigger my anxiety and send me running for the nearest bathroom to check and readjust my hair. Anyone who has experienced BDD will tell you of the terrifying consequences of different lighting, differently shaped mirrors, different angles, even the different expectations we bring with us to the mirror, all of which can smash our carefully constructed sense of safety into tiny pieces. I would often enter a bathroom, or any room with a mirror for that matter, feeling fine, exiting 10–30 minutes later as a different person: head down, eyes diverted, mumbling my words and feeling a weight of despair that had been brought on by a fluorescent lightbulb falling harshly on a cheekbone, or a warped mirror pinching my head at the temples. I imagine my friends would often wonder to themselves what on earth had happened to me while I was in there.

Soon enough, my behaviours were intruding on many aspects of my day-to-day life. This continued throughout my school days, across my time at university and into my working life as an adult. My first job was working as a teaching assistant in a lovely primary school. Throughout my day here, I would make excuses to go to the bathroom an unusual number of times, for an unusual amount of time, returning either unusually elated because I had managed to take a picture I liked, or unusually deflated because I had not. Eventually, this led to a complaint being made to the headmaster by the teacher I worked with, but I still did not disclose the underlying reason (I wouldn't like to attempt to remember the excuse I used at the time!).

In fact, I didn't really tell anyone about my BDD, certainly not my family, and I only dropped the smallest of hints to my girlfriend at the time. This made many of my behaviours difficult to understand for my loved ones: the hours I spent in the bathroom, the dozens of photos of myself on the family camera and the 'good ones' I had saved, simply suggesting I was unbelievably vain and self-obsessed, which was ironic given that this couldn't really be further from the truth. I would ask my girlfriend for regular reassurance and lived in fear of her rejecting me when she finally noticed the flaws I had so carefully kept hidden when we met. And so, I quietly dealt with BDD by myself, for years and years. Eventually, I became used to the BDD permeating and discolouring every aspect of my life, assuming and accepting there would never be a way out.

Obsession Put to Work

Before detailing my recovery from BDD, I would like to talk about the positive aspects that have come with the obsessive nature I have described. Although it led me down a path to developing BDD, I believe it has also been something of a superpower, providing me with an ability to laser-focus onto my interests and passions and develop skills I might not have been able to without it.

I have always been a highly creative person. From the age of ten, I learned multiple musical instruments, becoming proficient with the guitar, the drums, the piano and at singing. This was mostly because I could happily focus on practising for many hours at a time, something which often provided the bonus of a small alleviation of my BDD thoughts. I would also spend many hours drawing and painting. At the age of 18 I started attending art school (I was fascinated to later learn that 25 per cent of people experiencing BDD have a career or education in the arts) (Lambrou, Veale & Wilson, 2011). Here I became known for working on projects that others would have found maddening in their time-consuming meticulousness. Once, I painted a huge canvas entirely with the tip of a stretched-out paperclip. For a more sculptural piece, I made accurate cardboard cut-outs of all 200 countries in the world and placed them on a giant kebab skewer. I also recreated Van Gogh's famous *Starry Night Sky* with thousands of tiny eyes cut from fashion magazines, each one representing a brushstroke of the original oil painting. I'm sure you'll agree these are quite strange ideas, and I no longer remember my justification for creating them, but I think the main reason was because I *could*; I loved being consumed with the same repetitive task for hours, weeks and months at a time, and would gravitate towards ideas that would allow me to do so. Fortunately, the resulting images and objects were also quite striking in their level of minute detail. Just like when I practised a musical instrument, I could lose myself in activity, and my BDD would fade into the background for a while.

As a satisfied but somewhat unemployable art graduate, I began a career in education. Following ten years of working with children with various special educational needs, I eventually decided to pursue a career in educational psychology. This initially involved a conversion course at Bristol University. This was of course quite daunting; I had chosen to follow a career path I had no background in, with a view to gaining a place on a highly competitive funded doctoral course with only a hundred places nationwide, and over a thousand applicants. My one-in-ten shot was a long one, especially given that most applicants had already studied psychology for three years as part of an undergraduate course. I felt I had to give myself an edge. So, once again, I put my obsessive thought patterns to good use, fixating on the idea that I *had* to pass the course with the highest grade. Interestingly, I have a short attention span for most activities, but this can be completely overridden if my obsessive circuitry kicks into gear. Thus, I spent 12 hours each day reading textbooks, poring over research and writing my assignments. Once again, my obsessive mind had allowed me to latch on to an idea and hyper-focus on achieving something even I thought to be out of the question.

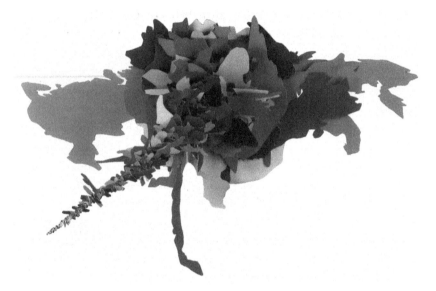

200 COUNTRIES ON A SKEWER

Although this hyper-focus has its benefits, it is not always a pleasant experience. I often still feel that hot, itchy feeling I had felt at the fairground as a child, the one that comes from feeling completely overwhelmed by an idea to the extent that I couldn't stop if I wanted to. It can come at the expense of everything else around me. If I'm in a state of hyper-focus, I find it difficult to stop to eat or even to use the toilet, and my social life can suffer as there isn't much space for anything else. If anyone else is in the room with me at these times (apologies to my girlfriend), an entire day can pass without a word from me, and interruptions can lead the hot, itchy feeling to spill over into undeserved irritation. I have had to become careful about what I let my mind latch on to, and I've had to minimise my music making because an unfinished song will not leave capacity in my head for the busy and demanding work of an educational psychologist.

It can sometimes be difficult to separate the behaviours that have allowed me to succeed from those which have caused me torment. In many ways, they are two sides of the same coin. Certainly, the line between them is often blurred. My artistic and creative side comes with a perfectionist streak: as a child, I would spend hours repetitively drawing cartoons, always featuring the same characters in the same positions, endlessly attempting to perfect their proportions. This reflects the hours spent in front of the mirror, desperately seeking a perfect symmetry in my face that almost no human truly has. At age ten, I began to learn to play the guitar and I often found it hard to make it beyond the first two bars of a piece of music I was learning, instead looping a small phrase, and practising until I could play it without any errors, however small. I can connect this to the way in which I used to focus in on the smallest detail of my own face, repeatedly examining it each time I looked into the mirror instead of looking at my face as a whole. Even now, I like to write and produce electronic music when I have the time, and I can all too easily spend hours on five seconds of music, played over and over and tweaked until it sounds just right to me. Even when I put my headphones down and walk away from my laptop, the music plays on in my mind and I find it hard to concentrate on anything else. At these times, I am reminded of stepping away from the mirror but only being afforded a few minutes of reprieve before the urge to look again grew too strong to resist.

In these ways, my obsessive nature often leads me to walk something of a knife's edge between advantageous and detrimental fixations. It's something I'm not entirely in control of and I've had to learn to harness it, like some bucking bronco that always threatens to throw me off its back. Mercifully, with time and effort, this can be achieved. So now I will talk about how I managed to tame my BDD.

Obsession Tamed

From the time my BDD began, to the age of around 25, I had not mentioned to a single soul the anxiety I was dealing with under the surface. This was partly because I found it embarrassing and shameful, and didn't want to draw attention to myself. It was also because I always assumed nobody could help me, besides perhaps a cosmetic surgeon.

I have theorised that this is the main reason why awareness of BDD is so low: people with BDD feel it is futile to seek help and may not be believed or understood if they do. I had dropped a few hints to my parents along the way, just to test the waters, but they had just dismissed it as a teenage phase. I don't blame them for this, as I imagine every teenager talks about disliking their appearance at one time or another, but the extra layer of preoccupation and intense anxiety make it quite a different experience for people experiencing BDD. 'Oh, don't worry about that darling, you look fine. Think about something else', my mum might say. Was it possible for other people to turn their thoughts off like that, like a tap? I came away from these moments ashamed of the anxiety I was experiencing, believing that stronger people were able to simply squash their negative thoughts about themselves and go about their lives happily. I told myself I was just being silly, but that didn't stop the anxiety gnawing away at me.

By the age of 25, the constant cloud of anxiety that was BDD had permeated my life for over a decade. I decided I wanted to be free of it, once and for all. The first step was a visit to the GP. When I described my symptoms, he looked through his medical manual and said, 'It sounds like you might have body dysmorphic disorder.' At this point, I had never actually heard the term before. So, on returning home I searched the internet for more information. Reading the diagnostic criteria gave me the uncanny feeling of having my mind read: they perfectly described what I had been dealing with. A preoccupation with my appearance? Certainly, barely a moment went by without it discolouring my thoughts. Repetitive behaviours relating to said preoccupation? Check. If I wasn't staring into the mirror or taking selfies and styling my hair, I was comparing myself to other people or otherwise ruminating on my appearance. Significant anxiety in response to all of this? Absolutely. BDD sometimes came at me in sharp peaks of intense panic, and although it was more often at a more manageable level, it was never absent. Discovering that my experience wasn't novel, that enough people experienced the same thing for it to have been given a fancy name in a diagnostic medical manual, was a revelation. This was the moment the seed of recovery was planted. A thought entered my head: *Perhaps this isn't to do with how I look; perhaps I need to change the way I think.* Although the thought was a fleeting one at this point, it was brand new, and it was a beam of light at the edge of an opening doorway.

I began to conduct more research into BDD, learning about how I might actually be able to overcome it. I had hope! I read about Cognitive

Behavioural Therapy (CBT), which involves challenging the negative cycles of thought and behaviour that perpetuate unnecessary anxiety. Could it be possible that I could *think* my way out of this?! I went back to the doctor and asked about how to put myself forward for this CBT. He referred me to a service offering ten free sessions with a trainee clinical psychologist, and so we began. The young psychologist was unfamiliar with BDD, but he listened carefully to my experiences and asked me questions which made me think in ways I hadn't before. In the presence of someone else, under a collaborative microscope, thoughts such as *I will never be loveable because of the shape of my head* can suddenly seem surprisingly disproportionate. The benefit of the sessions wasn't immediate, and in the short term I remember feeling worse. It was like digging up the soil, unearthing something that had been festering underground for a long time. At first, I was just making a real mess, flinging metaphorical mud over my shoulders. Yet somehow, after a while, it started to feel as though I had removed something unpleasant and was finally patting the soil back down into place.

Gradually, I realised that the BDD behaviours were starting to disappear. I would look into the mirror for less time. I would compare myself to other people less often and I would feel less concerned about my hair being in exactly the right position. This began to embolden me, and I started my own exposure therapy, having read that this was helpful for BDD also (it hadn't been part of the therapy itself, as it usually would be for BDD-specific CBT). This involved gradually cutting my own hair shorter by small amounts every few weeks, quite literally exposing the shape of my head to the world. Funnily enough, the final exposure came as an example of accidental flooding: I cut my hair so badly, I had to take a taxi to my friend's house, wearing a baseball cap and hiding my face, so she could fix it. My hair was now so short, choppy and lop-sided that she had to shave my head. This was one of the single most anxiety-inducing experiences of my life. What would people say when they saw me? What if they finally see my 'true' appearance and are horrified? Two halves of me wrestled with these thoughts – the CBT had weakened them, but they were certainly not dead. The next day I walked to the primary school I worked at with feelings of trepidation, and...nobody batted an eyelid.

'Oh wow, you shaved your head, it suits you!' they all said, in one variation or another, then carried on as if nothing had happened. No pointing, no laughing, no shocked looks. Almost instantly the last of my anxiety dissipated. My head was on full display for all the world to see, and this world hadn't collapsed around my ears. The last vestiges of my BDD thoughts were exposed to full daylight and could no longer hold up to scrutiny. This gave me such a feeling of freedom that I've kept a shaved head ever since, like a badge of honour. It's a constant reminder that I've achieved something I once thought was impossible, and vanquished the anxiety that had plagued me for so long.

I don't want to turn this narrative into too much of a fairytale, or to pretend all my problems were solved in this one moment. To this day, BDD is something I have to keep in check, and I feel there is always the possibility of relapse. Sometimes I will feel the pull of the mirror, or the camera lens, and I must resist the urge to check again. But the important thing I hold on to is that I can resist this urge. I can actually walk away and do something else, and that hot, itchy feeling goes away. Even more importantly, if I see a picture of myself that I don't like or catch myself at a bad angle in the mirror, I feel no anxiety whatsoever. This is what I see as true recovery from BDD. For me recovery is not about coming to love every aspect of the way I look, because I'm not sure anybody does. It's about learning to accept my flaws as nothing more than what makes me human. To feel a part of the human race, not some visiting alien, is more than enough for me.

And so, I have learned to accept and respect my obsessive nature. It has led me to some dark places, but it has also led me to overcome challenges. With time and effort, obsession can be harnessed and redirected in positive ways, which can eventually outweigh the negative spaces it can create in our minds, hearts and bodies. Interestingly, since overcoming my BDD, my other obsessive behaviours have fallen away alongside, and I no longer fixate *quite* so intensely on anything. I no longer have the energy to allow that hot, itchy feeling into my body, which may have something to do with age...though I also believe that having felt stillness in my mind and body provides me with the motivation to keep it that way.

To my fellow obsessives, and those working with them and supporting them, I would like to finish by saying that I think there is a reason for our existence. We have evolved to be the member of the tribe who can home in on details and examine things from the inside out. Just like more hyperactive personalities, who create and innovate by making huge leaps to connect far-flung dots, we are the quieter ones who examine and perfect those new forms of knowledge and invention. Obsession has a purpose. The invitation is to find out what this is! Importantly, helping clients to explore ways of harnessing aspects like attention to detail, local visual processing and hyper-focus as part of the therapeutic process can be richly beneficial when supporting people struggling with BDD.

Reference

Lambrou, C., Veale, D., & Wilson, G. (2011). The role of aesthetic sensitivity in body dysmorphic disorder. *Journal of Abnormal Psychology*, 120(2), 443.

Chapter 5

Considering Aspects of the Embodied Brain and Sensory System in the Experience of BDD

———

NICOLE SCHNACKENBERG

We experience the world through our senses. The brain interprets this sensory information, overlaying it at times with 'ghosts from the past' and present-moment perceptions of the self. This makes both the brain and sensory system essential considerations when working with body dysmorphic disorder (BDD), as we shall explore in this chapter. The chapter outlines relevant neuroscientific aspects of the three-part brain, the brain's left and right hemispheres, and global versus local processing, before moving on to a consideration of how sensory profiling can be supportive when working with people experiencing BDD.

There have been a number of neurological studies involving people diagnosed with BDD, from the first morphometric MRI (magnetic resonance imaging) study in 2003 conducted by Scott Rauch and colleagues, to more recent studies, for example looking at brain activation and connectivity patterns by Jamie Feusner and his research team in 2021 (Moody et al., 2021).

While many of these studies point to neurological nuances in BDD, they cannot, of course, ascertain whether these differences pre-existed (and therefore were a possibly precipitating factor in the emergence of) BDD and/or whether these differences were a *result* of the relational/ development trauma, distress, rumination, compulsive behaviours etc. characteristic of BDD. In the former case, we still cannot be sure why and how these differences emerged nor how any experiences/differences translate into the experience of BDD. The role of developmental trauma in the emerging architecture of the brain is, however, indisputable in empirical research (for a summary, see *Why Love Matters* by Sue Gerhardt (2014)). The same can be said of the impact of developmental trauma on the nervous and sensory systems also.

The Three-Part Brain and BDD

When working with people experiencing BDD, or indeed any emotional and mental health struggle, the three-part model of the brain can be useful to consider.

The brainstem is the area at the base of the brain that lies between cerebral hemispheres and the cervical spinal cord, sometimes colloquially referred to as the reptilian or primal brain. The brainstem regulates basic physiological processes such as the functioning of the heart and lungs and, thus, states of physiological arousal. It is also involved in the fight/flight/freeze/fawn response.

The brainstem is part of the motivational system towards getting basic needs met like eating, sleeping, keeping warm and feeling safe. A basic need that is sometimes overlooked, and one which is central to the experience of BDD, is that of connection: making relational, trusted and enjoyed connections with other human beings. If the threat-perception system is on high alert, as indeed it appears to be within the experience of BDD, the motivation to come close to and connect with others may be imbued with fear. Natalie Stechler explored this in more detail back in Chapter 3.

Next, we have the limbic system, a complex set of brain structures concerned with learning, memory and emotion. The limbic system operates by influencing the endocrine system and the autonomic nervous system. The amygdala, the deepest part of this limbic system, alerts us to possible dangers (real, perceived or imagined) in the internal and external environment. The amygdala, as we will read more about shortly, can ignite an instantaneous survival response. In the context of BDD, this appears to regularly be a 'flight' response, i.e. flighting to or from the mirror or other reflective surfaces; flighting from other people to negate potential rejection; flighting to a hat/scarf/make-up to camouflage the perceived defect etc.

Finally we have the outer layer of the brain, the cortex, implicated in self-awareness, imagination and cognitive thought processes. This part of the brain makes meta-cognition possible; the act of thinking about thinking and being aware of being aware. The prefrontal cortex, the area just behind the forehead, is the area within which representations of concepts are created, such as a sense of self, time and morality. Of course, the felt sense of self is central to the experience of BDD.

The Amygdala

The amygdala is an almond-shaped set of neurons located in the brain's medial temporal lobe. It plays an important part in emotions and behaviour and has an essential role in the processing of fear, and in the fear response. When one is exposed to a fearful stimulus, information about that stimulus is immediately sent to the amygdala which is then able to send signals to other areas of the brain to trigger a response, including the fight/flight/freeze/fawn response.

Pieces of information about fearful stimuli can reach the amygdala before one is consciously aware of them. Thus, a person can rapidly find themselves in a state of hyper-arousal, and indeed operating within a fear response, without knowing or understanding why or what triggered them. The amygdala receives inputs from all eight senses; vision, hearing, touch, taste, smell, proprioception, vestibular and interoception. Thus, one's felt sense of danger not only comes from input from the world around (exteroceptive) but also from input from the inside (interoceptive).

The amygdala is also central to the formation of emotion-related memories associated with both fear-inducing and reward-based events. Importantly, strong emotional memories (including those associated with fear and shame; again, central in the experience of BDD) are difficult to forget.

The amygdala is implicated in alerting one to danger and induces a cascade of physiological responses designed to mobilise a person to save themselves. The difficulty with an experience like BDD is that a person might be triggered continuously by stimuli they perceive and interpret (and which the amygdala perceives and interprets) as threatening which in fact are not objectively dangerous. Walking down the street, for example, a person might find themselves triggered by the sunlight (alongside fears this may accentuate their perceived flaws), people laughing while they socialise together (believing they are laughing at the perceived defect and/or the appearance more generally), physical sensations like heat and tingling in or around the perceived appearance flaw and so on. The amygdala and thus the sympathetic (energy mobilising) branch of the autonomic nervous system may go into overdrive, and the person may find themselves panicking without any clear sense of why they suddenly feel so afraid.

The amygdala can also be triggered by associations of past traumas, for example, bullying experiences. Indeed, research suggests that more people with a diagnosis of BDD have been bullied and have experienced these bullying experiences as more distressing, relative to the general population (e.g. Buhlmann et al., 2007).

The Hippocampus

The hippocampus is a complex brain structure which plays a major role both in memory and in the process of learning. Like the amygdala, it is also located in the medial temporal lobe of the brain. It has been suggested that it is via communication between the amygdala and the hippocampus – when emotion meets memory – that one can modify the recollection of events at will.

It is in the hippocampus that episodic memories are formed. Episodic memories are memories formed from events in one's life, like having lunch with a friend yesterday or, as we have mentioned, a bullying episode. While the hippocampus 'remembers' the details of the bullying experience the amygdala will 'remember' the emotional response. Thus, many of our clients with BDD may 'remember' emotionally rather than verbally, particularly if they have experienced developmental (and often pre-verbal) relational trauma, as many of them may have. The triggers for their distress, therefore, may be beneath the level of conscious, verbal awareness. For example, the person may find themselves picking at their skin suddenly without knowing what caused them to feel unsafe or anxious.

The hippocampus is vital not only for learning and memory but also for spatial navigation. Visual-spatial awareness in BDD is another area of interest. Anomalies in visual processing systems, including visuospatial anomalies, have been identified in people diagnosed with BDD in some of the neuroscientific studies (e.g. Feusner et al., 2011). This includes a propensity towards local (small detail) as opposed to global processing. You will have read in the last chapter about how Alex, who is an expert-by-lived-experience of BDD and also a psychologist, would paint pictures with the end of a paperclip and other such pursuits, highlighting this local processing propensity poignantly.

Left and Right Hemispheres

The human brain is divided into two hemispheres – the left and the right – connected by the corpus callosum in the centre. The left hemisphere processes sensory inputs from the right side of the body while the right hemisphere processes sensory inputs from the left side of the body. The two hemispheres have an inhibitory function on one another via this corpus callosum, which is full of inhibitory neurons. It is necessary to inhibit one hemisphere in order to inhabit the other, e.g. to inhibit local processing (left hemisphere) to engage in global processing (right hemisphere).

The left hemisphere of the brain is concerned with logic and linearity and leans towards black-and-white ways of seeing the world. Interestingly, in 95–97 per cent of the population, language is localised to this left hemisphere. The right hemisphere, on the other hand, is concerned with the emotional life of the human being including the phenomenon of interoception: the lived experience of the body from the inside. This includes awareness of signals like body temperature, heart rate, breathing rate, blood pressure, pain, hunger and fullness, and sexual arousal.

One of the most fundamental differences between the hemispheres is the type of attention they give to the world. The left hemisphere pays focused attention (local processing) while the right hemisphere applies broad scope (global) processing. This is highly relevant to the experience of BDD as people experiencing BDD tend to process visual information locally as opposed to globally – to home in on intricacies within their visual field – and are often described as having 'an eye for detail' (e.g. Feusner, Yaryura-Tobias & Saxena, 2008).

Interestingly, the left hemisphere of the brain focuses on what it already knows, while the right hemisphere is open to new information. The left hemisphere, therefore, is predictive rather than curious. It 'sees' what it expects to see. The left hemisphere is, as a result, not efficient at revising initial assumptions or at distinguishing new information from old information.

The right hemisphere presents an array of possible solutions, unlike the left, which takes a solution that seems to best fit what it already knows and latches on to it, ignoring any discrepancies in the process. Therefore, inhabiting the right hemisphere of the brain can also support taking on new and alternative views of reality to those already held. This can be beneficial in the experience of BDD within which there is a propensity to become 'stuck' in the so-perceived reality of a supposed appearance defect or flaw. This can also support the process of taking a longer-term view of one's behaviours, experiences and difficulties rather than a short-term view (another of the propensities of the left hemisphere).

In addition, it is interesting to note that the left hemisphere tends to be preoccupied by anxious apprehension, based on a fear of uncertainty and a sense of a lack of control. The fear of uncertainty and unpredictability often go very much hand in hand with the experience of BDD. It is typical for a person experiencing BDD to struggle with how aspects of their appearance seem to alter and shift from mirror to mirror, hour to hour and even minute to minute. People experiencing BDD often live in dread of noticing another blemish, seeing another shift in the shape of their nose and so on.

Differentially to the left hemisphere, the right hemisphere is less preoccupied with the future and has a greater capability of staying in the present moment. It is also more open and flexible to change and uncertainty.

Global Processing and 'Open Attention'

The right hemisphere is responsible for all types of attention aside from focused attention (the primary type of attention applied in BDD). Naturally, the way in which one pays attention to the world alters the way one perceives and experiences the world. The world one experiences in any given moment is determined by which hemisphere's version of the world is predominating. While inhabiting the left hemisphere of the brain, one is likely to perceive the appearance piecemeal and to focus in on perceived flaws and defects. Therefore, supporting our clients to inhabit the right hemisphere of the brain can be beneficial. Some ideas for prompting greater inhabitation of the right hemisphere of the brain include:

- Listening to music played in a minor key.

- Creative and artistic pursuits.

- Reading or writing poetry.

- Tuning into interoceptive signals such as the heartbeat, the breathing pattern, sensations of heat or coolness in the body etc.

- Moving the left side of the body.

- Writing, drawing, painting etc. with the left hand (or foot).

- Blocking the right nostril and breathing for a few breath cycles through the left nostril.

A practice I often use with clients experiencing BDD, and one which regularly invites profound insights, is to invite them to ask a question of their BDD with their right hand (thus, the left hemisphere); then to take a moment (with their hands on their heart if this feels comfortable for them) to allow an answer to bubble up (inviting the thinking part of their brain to relax); then to place the pen/pencil/crayon etc. into the left hand and write the answer onto the page (from the right hemisphere). Some of the questions clients have found helpful to pose to BDD include:

- Why did you come into my life?

- What are you afraid of?

- How can I help you to relax?

- How old do you think I am? (The BDD part often thinks the person is considerably younger than their chronological age, i.e. the age of an infant or young child.)

For a more detailed description of exploring BDD through different parts/aspects of the self, please see Chapter 13 outlining some potential uses of the Voice Dialogue approach for BDD. *The Power of the Other Hand: A Course in Channelling the Inner Wisdom of the Right Brain* by Lucia Capacchione (1988) is also recommended when exploring this and similar approaches.

Egocentric and Allocentric Attention

Attention can be categorised into two distinct functions: bottom-up attention and top-down attention. Bottom-up attention is attention driven purely by external factors while top-down attention refers to an internal guidance of attention based on prior knowledge and goals.

Alongside these two functions of attention, there are two main ways in which one visually perceives reality. These are contingent on the way attention is paid. The first is the egocentric processing system. When we look at an object from this mode of processing, photons from that object are transformed by the eye into impulses relayed to the brain. The brain then represents the object's visual image in three-dimensional spatial coordinates. This 'object message' is referred directly back to brain circuits representing the physical self. Thus, the somatic self remains the central axis receiving this self-referent 3D perception. The object perceived is automatically a self-centred, egocentric reconstruction of the object. The sense is one of, *I am a unique someone who is looking at that object over there.* This 'object' could be the self or an aspect of the self perceived in the mirror.

The vantage point for this mode of perception is from the left hemisphere of the brain. This egocentric processing pathway overlaps with the two major modules for top-down visual processing: the intraparietal sulcus and the frontal eye field, flowing first through the parietal lobe. This implies that the top-down form of attentive processing is inherently linked with the processing of the personal, physical self (somatic self). In the parietal lobe, two highly personal senses are enlisted: proprioception (the sense of the body in space), and the sense of touch.

Importantly, there is a second way of perceiving reality, one we might be less aware of and accustomed to. This mode of perception is other-centred and often referred to as *allocentric* perception (from the Greek *allos*, meaning 'other'). Allocentric perception describes an externalised perspective that creates images of objects in the outside world. The object seen through this mode is seen to co-exist in relation to other objects 'out there', not in reference to one's somatic being as felt to be in the centre.

Unlike the egocentric stream, the allocentric stream flows through networks in the temporal lobe. It is accessible to the two other modules of attention that serve bottom-up attentive functions: the temporo-parietal junction and the inferior frontal cortex. These temporal lobe networks are designed for making meaningful interpretations based on what is seen and heard.

Egocentric representations of objects are proposed to underlie goal-directed actions while allocentric representations are proposed to support the conscious perception of objects. Could it be that in BDD, the person is objectifying the body and processing this body-object egocentrically, with the goal-directed action being to alter or fix the perceived defect in some way? If this is the case, exploring the possibility of processing the visual of the body allocentrically may support our clients in consciously perceiving the body in the present moment, as opposed to as an object overlaid with painful memories from the past and projected desires for the future. Inhabiting the right hemisphere of the brain would, again, be supportive of this process.

Clients may use different attentional 'hooks' to anchor them in the present moment and support allocentric processing, such as focusing on the breath or on an object like a flower, a cloud, a single note within a piece of music or the flickering flame of a candle. In fact, any of the senses can be called upon for these anchors. Supporting our clients to increase their understanding of their sensory profile and related propensities can be beneficial to this process.

Sensory Profiling

Each of us has a unique sensory profile. The way we process the world through our senses may be affected by a range of phenomena including psychobiological factors, early life experiences and medical history. It is possible to experience hyper-(over-)arousal in some of the senses in all or some situations, and hypo-(under-)arousal in some or all situations in other senses. It is also possible to uncomfortably oscillate between hyper-arousal and hypo-arousal within the same sense.

Supporting our clients to better understand their sensory profile can facilitate an increase in self-awareness and understanding; help them to ascertain potent anchors for present-moment allocentric awareness; aid them in finding ways of balancing the autonomic nervous system (please see Chapter 8); and invite a discovery of therapeutic modalities and approaches best matched to their proclivities. You might like to encourage and support your client to complete the sensory profiles offered throughout the rest of this chapter, which have been adapted from the work of Olga Bogdashina (2016), and then to explore practices and approaches related to each aspect of their profile together with them.

Some clients may complete the profiles within therapeutic sessions alongside yourself, while others may fill them out at home later and bring them to sessions for discussion and reflection. Either way, it is useful to explore each of the eight senses steadily in turn, rather than trying to fit every sense into a single session, allowing for a rich, in-depth discussion of how any hypo- or hyper-sensitivities may play out within your client's BDD and life more generally. This can then lead to a consideration of what sensory adaptations can be made to their day-to-day lives, alongside exploring which practices and techniques may be the most regulating and soothing.

Sensory Profile: Vision

	Yes ✓ No ✗
Vision	
I struggle to recognise a familiar environment if approached from a different direction	☐
I select for attention minor aspects of objects rather than the whole thing	☐
I have difficulties with judging spatial relationships	☐
I get lost easily	☐
I am startled when approached suddenly	☐
Hyper	
I tend to notice every visual change in the environment	☐
I am easily distracted by visual stimuli in the environment	☐
I tend to be captivated by minute particles, pieces of fluff etc.	☐
I keep 'seeing' a visual stimulus after it has gone	☐
I dislike bright lights	☐
I am frightened by sharp flashes of light	☐
I fear heights, stairs, escalators; I hesitate going up and down steps	☐
I look down a lot of the time	☐
I cover or close my eyes or squint at bright light	☐
I often avoid eye contact	☐
I have a good visual memory	☐
Hypo	
I am attracted to lights	☐
I tend to look intensely at objects/people	☐
I am fascinated with reflections/bright objects	☐
I like to run my hands around the edges of an object	☐
I like to touch items in a room to get a sense of where I am	☐
I don't recognise people in unfamiliar clothes	☐
My response to visual stimuli is often delayed (e.g. I fail to close my eyes when a light is suddenly switched on)	☐

Adapted from Bogdashina (2016)

People with visual sensitivities alongside a propensity for local rather than global processing (both very common in BDD) are often interested in fine art, editing and other related pursuits, as indeed many people with BDD are. There are a multitude of art-focused practices your clients may feel drawn towards and find helpful. Here are just a few ideas.

OBSERVING A PIECE OF ART MINDFULLY

From viewing art in an art gallery or looking at pieces online, it can be a lovely practice to stay with a single artwork for an extended period of time rather than using that period of time to look at multiple pieces. Your client might benefit from popping into a gallery, for example, for ten minutes to spend time looking at one painting or one sculpture. Encourage your client to allow themselves to zoom in and out, directing their gaze to aspects of the piece and to the piece as a whole. If they notice judgments coming into their mind about the piece, they could try noticing these judgments then redirecting their focus and attention back to witnessing the piece allocentrically in the present moment, exactly as it is.

KALEIDOSCOPE

Sinking one's attention into the shifting patterns and colours of a kaleidoscope can be a very mindful and soothing practice.

STAR-GAZING

Looking up into a night sky can support a sense of awe, wonder and perspective. This can be done with the naked eye or with a telescope. It can also be enjoyable to have a go at identifying and tracing constellations with the eye-gaze, perhaps even drawing the constellations into a little sketchbook for future reference.

TRATAKA/CANDLE-GAZING

Trataka is a visual form of meditation in the yogic tradition, wherein the open eyes are focused on a small point or object. Frequently, Trataka is practised with a candle, with the attention focused on the flame.

The person finds a quiet and (if they feel comfortable) a darkened space where, ideally, they will not be disturbed. It is a good idea to leave mobile phones and any other distractions in another room. Place the candle at the level of the eye gaze and light it. Find a comfortable seated position, taking a cardigan or shawl around the shoulders if needed as the body temperature is likely to drop as the body is brought to stillness.

It is ideal to sit about two feet away from the candle and bring the eye gaze to gently rest on the flame. Sink the attention and awareness as completely as possible into the image of the flickering flame. Hold the eyes steady, blinking naturally, and gently bring them back to the flame if the eyes wander elsewhere. At the end of whatever time period has been chosen for this practice, the person might like to lie down (or remain sitting if this feels more comfortable) and close their eyes. They may or may not have the visual image of the candle flame continue to flicker for a while in their mind's eye.

I have also found small plants or stones to be beautiful focal points for the practice of Trataka.

MINDFUL READING

In this practice, a sentence or a short piece of prose or a poem is taken and read very slowly, perhaps putting an inhalation and an exhalation between each word. Your client could be encouraged to choose something that soothes, uplifts and/or inspires them.

Another option is for your client to take a short piece of text written in a language they do not speak or understand. This allows the mind to bypass any struggle or associations with the meaning of the words and, rather, to sink the awareness into the visual of the words written on the page and the sound of their rhythm and cadence (particularly if read aloud), making it, also, a more right hemisphere activity and experience. I personally like to read in Gurmukhi, an ancient Indian poetic language.

VISUALISATION

There are many guided visualisations your client might like to try on the various available mindfulness apps and on the internet. Your client can also create their own simple visualisations, for example:

- Visualising a safe, calming place to which they can go at any time in their mind's eye, e.g. a beach, a forest or a cosy room.

- Bringing to mind the face of a supportive loved one.

- Visualising oneself undertaking a feared action with a calm heart, e.g. going into a crowded shop.

- Visualising images of hope such as a flower opening slowly to the sunlight, a sunrise, a rainbow, a butterfly emerging from a chrysalis etc.

Sensory Profile: Hearing

	Yes ✓ / No ✗
Hearing	
I struggle to concentrate in a crowded, noisy room	☐
I don't seem to understand instructions if more than one person is talking	☐
I keep 'hearing' the sound after it has been switched off/stops	☐
I tend to hear (with meaning) a few words rather than the whole sentence	☐
I have sound/word pronunciation difficulties	☐
I am often unable to distinguish between some sounds	☐
My response to some sounds is delayed	☐
Hyper	
I tend to cover my ears at some sounds	☐
I experience some sounds as painful	☐
I am a light sleeper	☐
I dislike thunderstorms, crowds etc.	☐
I avoid some sounds/noises	☐
I am distracted by sounds others are unaware of	☐
I sometimes make repetitive noises to myself to block out other sounds	☐
I have a good auditory memory	☐
Hypo	
I tend to bang objects, doors	☐
I like vibrations	☐
I like excessively loud music, TV etc.	☐
I am attracted by sounds/noises	☐
I am fascinated with certain sounds	☐

Adapted from Bogdashina (2016)

Developmental trauma and other traumas such as bullying can leave a person with palpable auditory sensitivities of various kinds. For example, they may be hyper-sensitive to loud voices, to voices with certain tones and pitches, to laughter and so on. Hyper-vigilance can also lead to hearing every sound in the environment and finding it difficult to filter out foreground sounds (such as someone speaking) from background sounds (such as the hum of the refrigerator). The following practices focused on the auditory sense may be helpful.

MINDFUL LISTENING TO AUDIOBOOKS, PODCASTS ETC.

It is worth supporting your client to take the time to find a reader with a voice of a pitch, prosody and cadence that feels soothing and reassuring to them. The optimal pitch of human voice can be incredibly regulating. Mindful listening differs from a more general type of listening by virtue of the way in which one applies full attention to the sound of the voice, rather than listening while doing something else. If the mind wanders, the person can gently lead it back to the auditory input without judgment.

MINDFUL LISTENING TO MUSIC

Music tuned to 432 Hz is softer and brighter, providing more clarity of sound (hertz, Hz, is the unit of frequency). People have reported experiencing more meditative and relaxing states of mind and body when listening to music tuned to this frequency (Halbert et al. 2018). Due to its greater clarity, there is less requirement to play pieces of music at 432 Hz as loudly, resulting in reduced noise pressure. Verdi and Mozart are examples of composers for music played at this pitch. There have now also been many pieces of meditative music created at this frequency. Listening mindfully to music played at this pitch may, therefore, support clients to come into a state of relaxed awareness.

As mentioned earlier in the chapter, the right hemisphere of the brain is particularly awakened by music played in a minor key.

MINDFUL LISTENING TO NATURE

There are many possibilities here such as sinking one's awareness into the sound of birdsong, a trickling stream, the waves of the ocean, the rustle of leaves in the wind and so on.

LISTENING TO THOUGHTS ALOUD

This can be a particularly useful practice for increasing awareness and space around cyclical, self-negating thoughts. One option is for your client to audio-record themselves speaking their thoughts out loud, initially perhaps for a couple of minutes, then building up to longer periods of time as they become more comfortable with the process. Your client can then sit or lie down in a relaxed position, inviting the breath to be long and deep, and listen to the recording back, perhaps directing their attention more to the sound of the voice than the content of the thoughts themselves.

HUMMING BEE BREATH

Humming bee breath stimulates the vagus nerve, a parasympathetic (rest and digest) nerve which runs down the back of the throat and wanders throughout the body. One inhales deeply through the nose then hums the breath out, with closed lips, on the exhalation, humming all the way to the end of the exhalation before taking an inhalation through the nose and repeating the cycle. The awareness may be placed onto the sound of the self humming.

Sensory Profile: Touch

	Yes ✓ No ✗
Tactility	
I am unable to distinguish between tactile stimuli of different intensities (e.g. light and firm touch)	☐
I keep feeling a tactile sensation after it has ended	☐
I insist on wearing the same clothes	☐
I find nail cutting distressing/painful	☐
I feel discomfort from parts of clothes, e.g. labels	☐
Some parts of my body are hyper-sensitive to touch while others are hypo-sensitive	☐
I tend to pick at my skin, pull at my hair, hit myself etc. when distressed	☐
My response to tactile stimuli is sometimes delayed	☐
I sometimes hear sounds and/or see colours when I am touched	☐
Hyper	
As a baby, I didn't like to be held or cuddled	☐
I often resist being touched	☐
I find it distressing to wear new or stiff clothing	☐
I am often distressed by clothes, seams etc. rubbing on the skin	☐

Some aspects of self-care are painful to me, e.g. brushing the teeth and hair, taking a shower ☐

I often overreact to cold, heat, pain etc. ☐

I am disgusted by foods of certain textures ☐

I have a high gag reflex (food of certain textures) ☐

I tend to avoid standing in close proximity to others ☐

I have a good tactile memory ☐

Hypo

I like tactile pressure and tight clothing ☐

I hug and shake hands tightly ☐

I am not bothered by cuts and bruises ☐

I have a low reaction to pain and temperature ☐

I am prone to self-injury ☐

I am unable to distinguish which body part was touched if I am not looking ☐

I often struggle to interpret tactile sensations ☐

Adapted from Bogdashina (2016)

Touch is incredibly important to human beings, so much so that psychoanalyst Alessandra Lemma refers to the infant–caregiver relationship as the touch–gaze relationship (Lemma, 2010). Thus, stimulating the pressure receptors on our skin can be very soothing. Here are a few ideas of simple practices you might like to suggest to your clients.

SQUEEZING DOWN THE ARMS AND LEGS
Your client takes one of their hands and applies deep pressure to the top of their other arm by squeezing firmly. They hold for a few seconds, or as long as feels good in their body. They then continue all the way down the arm, squeezing also the fingers when they get there, before repeating with the other hand/arm. All the while, it can be supportive to breathe deeply.

This same practice can be applied to each leg in turn, squeezing gradually all the way down to the toes and also giving the toes a deep squeeze. If squeezing doesn't feel good in their body, your client might like to try flickering their fingers down each opposite arm and down the legs – a bit like heavy/firm raindrops.

SELF-MASSAGE OF THE HANDS AND/OR FEET

We have multiple acupressure points in the hands and feet. Massaging these can induce a relaxation response. If your client is interested in this approach, they may like to research the proposed benefits of the various acupressure points in the hands and feet and to have a go at massaging these. For example, the hand valley point is proposed to help reduce stress as well as alleviate shoulder tension and neck pain. Trialling reflexology and/or massage sessions with a qualified practitioner may be beneficial also.

Sensory Profile: Smell and Taste

	Yes ✓ No ✗
Olfaction (smell)	
I am unable to distinguish between strong and weak odours	☐
I tend to have a prolonged perception of olfactory stimuli	☐
My response to smells is often delayed	☐
I have difficulty interpreting smells	☐
Hyper	
I often complain about strong smells others do not notice	☐
I struggle to eat some foods because of their smell	☐
I am bothered by the smell of cooking	☐
I like to wear the same clothes because of the way they smell	☐
I cannot tolerate some smells/am nauseated by some odours	☐
Hypo	
I like to smell myself, people and objects	☐
I seek strong odours	☐
I don't seem to smell odours	☐

Adapted from Bogdashina (2016)

Taste/Gustation

Yes ✓
No ×

I am unable to distinguish between bland and spicy food ☐

I have a prolonged perception of taste ☐

My response to taste is delayed ☐

The taste of some foods causes me emotional distress ☐

Hyper

I am a picky eater ☐

I only eat bland foods ☐

I am careful to only use the tip of my tongue for tasting ☐

I gag/vomit easily ☐

I often experience a non-existent taste in my mouth ☐

I have a good memory for taste ☐

Hypo

I will eat anything ☐

I lick/eat inedible objects sometimes ☐

I crave excessively salty, spicy, sour foods ☐

I am fascinated with certain tastes ☐

Adapted from Bogdashina (2016)

Taste and smell might not instantly seem like obvious phenomena for practices to soothe the experience of BDD, yet for some people they will be extremely effective 'attentional hooks' and invitations to the right hemisphere of the brain. Here are some ideas you might like to try with your clients.

MINDFUL EXPLORATION OF THE SPICE CUPBOARD

Go into the kitchen or wherever the spices are kept. Select a few items which have distinct smells such as oregano, paprika, ginger, cumin and so on. Take time to place each spice under the nose in turn, taking a few deep breaths before moving on to the next spice. Sink the awareness into the sensations which arise as the scent of each spice is taken in. This activity may prompt reflection on a life event or person given how strongly the olfactory sense is connected to memory.

OLFACTORY-FOCUSED WALK IN NATURE

Take a walk outside with your client, perhaps in a park or forest, or maybe they would like to try this alone. Focus the attention on the smells arising. If the mind wanders to thoughts about other things, gently lead it back to the sensation of smelling. It can also be helpful to silently label each smell as it comes into awareness to focus the attention and bring the mind into the present moment, e.g. *tree sap, grass, blossom, earth.*

MINDFUL EATING

Vietnamese Buddhist teacher Thich Nhat Hanh suggests using an apple to practise a mindful eating meditation (of course, your client can select another food if apples are not pleasing and/or indigestible for them). You might like to share the following guidance with your client:

> Sit quietly, without any distractions such as watching the television or browsing the internet. Give your full attention to the apple, taking time to notice the apple's characteristics. You might notice the colour of the apple, how it feels in the hands, what it smells like and so on. Once you have taken time to examine the apple, take a bite. Chew slowly, placing the full light of your attention on the taste, the sensations of chewing and swallowing, and your reactions to the process. If your mind wanders, keep leading it back to the sensations associated with the apple. Continue to eat the apple with this focused awareness until it is finished.

Sensory Profile: Proprioception

Proprioception	Yes ✓ No ✗
Others describe me as clumsy and/or I tend to move stiffly	
I have prolonged perception of proprioceptive sensations	
I often complain about painful limbs	
I have difficulty with buttons, laces, getting dressed etc.	
I have poor body awareness (I bump into things easily)	
I have poor gross and fine motor skills	
I have difficulty learning dance movements	
I have difficulties with chewing, sucking, swallowing	

Hyper

People say I place my body in strange positions ☐

I have difficulty manipulating small objects ☐

I regularly turn my whole body to look at something ☐

I tend to walk on my toes ☐

I cannot tolerate certain body postures ☐

I experience non-existent body experiences, e.g. *It feels like I am flying* ☐

Hypo

I have poor muscle tone ☐

I have a weak grasp/drop things easily ☐

I have a lack of awareness of my body position in space ☐

I often appear floppy; I often lean against furniture etc. ☐

I stumble and fall frequently ☐

I tend to chew on pens and similar objects ☐

I grind my teeth ☐

I often rock back and forth ☐

I have difficulty in copying movements ☐

Adapted from Bogdashina (2016)

Repetitive, rhythmic, patterned and predictable movement is naturally soothing to the brainstem. This could include walking, jogging, dancing, skipping, jumping on a rebound trampoline, playing a musical instrument, knitting, sweeping the floor and so on.

Breath-led practices such as yoga and Qi Gong can be particularly beneficial. Here are a few related activities your client may wish to try.

MINDFUL WALKING

Mindful walking has been used as a technique for thousands of years. There are many ways of going about walking mindfully; the suggestion laid out here is just one idea you might like to share with your client:

Choose an area you can easily walk up and down or around in a circuit without being disturbed. This might be a place in nature or might simply be walking backwards and forwards across your living room. Begin by placing your awareness on the sensations on the soles of your feet. Lift up one foot, saying 'lifting' to yourself as you do so. Take a slow step, saying 'placing' to yourself as you place your foot down onto the earth. Continue like this, focusing your attention on and labelling each lift of the foot and each placing of the foot. If the mind wanders, gently bring it back to the lifting and placing, and to the sensations in the soles of the feet as you do so.

5RHYTHMS MOVEMENT OR FREE-STYLE DANCE

5Rhythms is a movement meditation practice which was devised by dancer Gabrielle Roth in the 1970s. The five rhythms danced are *flowing*, *staccato*, *chaos*, *lyrical* and *stillness*. There are many videos online of Gabrielle Roth and other practitioners describing the process, and classes are available across many parts of the globe.

Alternatively, your client might simply like to put on a piece of music and move the body mindfully in rhythm with the music. They can allow themselves to move spontaneously, placing their awareness onto the impulse to move and the lived expression of each movement. For some clients, dance practices or classes with clear steps may feel more containing and soothing than free-style approaches, particularly initially.

Sensory Profile: Vestibular

	Yes ✓ No ✗
Vestibular	
I resist changes to my head position/body movement/new motor activities	☐
I have a prolonged perception of vestibular stimuli	☐
I fear heights, stairs, escalators	☐
I tend to hold my head upright when leaning forwards or bending over	☐
I am unable to change body position to accommodate the task	☐
I have poor balance	☐
I tend to think in movements	☐
Hyper	
I have fearful reactions to normal movement activities	☐
I have strong difficulties with walking on uneven surfaces	☐
I strongly dislike my head being upside down	☐

I avoid lifts and escalators ☐

I am terrified of falling ☐

I become anxious when my feet leave the ground ☐

I experience movement sensations while still ☐

I become easily disorientated and dizzy ☐

Hypo

I continually seek out movement activities ☐

I have always enjoyed swings, see-saws etc. ☐

I like spinning around ☐

I crave intense rides at amusement parks ☐

I am always on the move ☐

I often rock back and forth without realising it ☐

I frequently put my head upside down ☐

I have low safety awareness ☐

Adapted from Bogdashina (2016)

Simple movements can stimulate and/or soothe the vestibular system. Here are a few ideas.

ROCKING

One can simply rock back and forth while seated, placing the awareness on the sensations in the body as one rocks: a rocking chair or a swing can be used. You might like to support your client to experiment with inhaling as they rock backwards and exhaling as they rock forwards. They can also lie on a yoga mat, bend the knees into the chest and rock backwards and forwards along the length of the spine. Rocking and swaying from leg to leg while standing is another option.

SPINNING

You may have heard of Sufi whirling, a form of movement meditation founded by Rumi in the 13th century. First, one stands with the right arm crossed over the left with the hands gently resting on the shoulders. The invitation is then to bow down to whatever one reveres the most, before standing and lifting the arms, right arm up with the palm facing up and the left arm down with the palm facing down while one spins around.

If your client has vestibular hyper-sensitivities, this may not be the practice for them as it may leave them feeling nauseous and uncomfortably disorientated. However, people with vestibular hypo-sensitivities can find this a very grounding, soothing and uplifting practice.

Sensory Profile: Interoception

	Yes ✓ No ✗
Interoception	
I have differential awareness of bodily sensations	☐
I tend to have poor self-care, e.g. may not eat enough or consume too much food in one sitting	☐
I have a propensity to go out in cold weather without enough clothing	☐
Hyper	
I experience temperature and other tactile inputs as painful	☐
I have a strong reaction to pain experiences	☐
I have a strong emotional response to hunger and/or fullness signals	☐
I often seek dark, quiet spaces	☐
I have a painful/strong awareness of my heartbeat	☐
I regularly feel I am hyperventilating	☐
Hypo	
I do not notice when I am hungry or full	☐
I have poor detection of temperature and pain	☐
I regularly feel numb and disconnected from the world and others	☐
I seek out strong sensation-based experiences, e.g. spicy foods, extreme temperatures	☐
I have a high pain threshold/do not notice injuries	☐

Adapted from Bogdashina (2016)

Interoceptive signals are sensations which are the result of interoceptors, or sensory nerve receptors, that receive and transmit sensations from stimuli originating in the interior of the body. The capacity to feel and process these sensations sits alongside the capacity to sense and process emotions.

People struggling with BDD have typically learnt to deny, fear and/or suppress the sensations in their body for any number of reasons such as traumatic relational experiences. In the process, they may have become cut off from their interoceptive signals (and emotional lives) and may describe a feeling of 'deadness' in the body and a sense of being 'disconnected from the neck down'.

Encouragingly, neuroscientists recognise that people can and do improve their knowledge of interoceptive stimuli. Yoga and other mindful movement practices are one way of supporting interoceptive awareness, with yoga mentioned by numerous authors as beneficial in chapters within this book (for example Anna Warhurst (Chapter 1), Jill Lubienski (7) and Jo Dance (6)).

There are many forms of yoga. It is worth noting that certain practices may be more beneficial to some clients, while other practices are better suited for others. If your client is prone to anxiety and states of sympathetic hyper-arousal, slower rhythmic practices may be soothing for them, such as Yin yoga. If they tend towards low mood and apathy, a more vigorous practice may be supportive, such as Vinyasa flow or Kundalini yoga. Your client may benefit from trying out different classes to find a practice that best suits them.

I recommend encouraging your clients to seek out yoga teachers who have undertaken additional training in yoga therapy, mental health and trauma-informed, trauma-sensitive practice. If attending a class feels too difficult for your client, many yoga therapists in particular offer one-to-one sessions which they can tailor to specific needs. There are also now many platforms and classes available online.

Concluding Reflections

Increasing our understanding of the brain and sensory system as therapists, and sharing this information with our clients, can be supportive in the context of BDD. Since BDD appears to predominantly 'operate' from the left hemisphere of the brain, sharing right-brained practices, in line with the nuances of each client's particular sensory profile, can support sensory soothing, emotional connection and regulation, and a fresh perspective on one's appearance, sense of self and the world.

Completing a sensory profile with our clients can offer prompts for rich discussion and a consideration of the breadth of factors impacting on their lived, embodied experience of BDD.

References

Bogdashina, O. (2016). *Sensory perceptual issues in autism and Asperger syndrome: Different sensory experiences – different perceptual worlds*. Jessica Kingsley Publishers.

Buhlmann, U., Cook, L. M., Fama, J. M., & Wilhelm, S. (2007). Perceived teasing experiences in body dysmorphic disorder. *Body Image, 4*(4), 381–385.

Capacchione, L. (1988). *The power of the other hand: A course in channelling the inner wisdom of the right brain*. Newcastle.

Feusner, J. D., Hembacher, E., Moller, H., & Moody, T. D. (2011). Abnormalities of object visual processing in body dysmorphic disorder. *Psychological Medicine, 41*(11), 2385–2397.

Feusner, J. D., Yaryura-Tobias, J., & Saxena, S. (2008). The pathophysiology of body dysmorphic disorder. *Body Image, 5*(1), 3–12.

Gerhardt, S. (2014). *Why love matters: How affection shapes a baby's brain*. Routledge.

Halbert, J. D., van Tuyll, D. R., Purdy, C., Hao, G., et al. (2018). Low Frequency Music Slows Heart Rate and Decreases Sympathetic Activity. *Music and Medicine, 10*(4), 180–185.

Lemma, A. (2010). *Under the skin: A psychoanalytic study of body modification*. Routledge.

Moody, T. D., Morfini, F., Cheng, G., Sheen, C. L., Kerr, W. T., Strober, M., & Feusner, J. D. (2021). Brain activation and connectivity in anorexia nervosa and body dysmorphic disorder when viewing bodies: Relationships to clinical symptoms and perception of appearance. *Brain Imaging and Behaviour, 15*(3), 1235–1252.

Rauch, S. L., Phillips, K. A., Segal, E., Makris, N., Shin, L. M., Whalen, P. J., ... & Kennedy, D. N. (2003). A preliminary morphometric magnetic resonance imaging study of regional brain volumes in body dysmorphic disorder. *Psychiatry Research: Neuroimaging, 122*(1), 13–19.

Chapter 6

BDD, Yoga and the Overall Direction of Travel

———

JO DANCE

I have never actually been given a formal diagnosis of body dysmorphic disorder (BDD), but I think it's fair to say I have the condition (with an awareness that labels can be both helpful and limiting and are perhaps best used as starting points for exploration). Thankfully, the BDD thoughts I experience seem to be on the milder end of the spectrum. They haven't prevented me from leaving the house, for example, but they still impact me in numerous ways. In this chapter I will explore what has been most helpful to me in my personal journey through BDD, particularly the practice of yoga including breathwork and meditation.

Looking back, I started developing the first signs of BDD when I was about 12 years old, if not earlier. It wasn't really surprising, considering I'd spent much of my life up until then in leotards with coaches who were regularly verbally abusive and overly critical. I went on to train full-time in dance from the age of 13, spending much of my time surrounded by mirrors. The often high-pressure world of ballet further developed the anxieties about my appearance.

As a younger child, I experienced uncomfortable eczema in a few places on my body. After trying countless steroid creams and other conventional treatments, in desperation I was taken to a family friend who was an experienced naturopath and was able to help clear it up in a matter of weeks. But in my early teens, it returned, just at the time when I was starting to feel more self-conscious about my appearance. As if by a cruel twist of fate, instead of being in the discreet places it was before, the eczema had moved to my face, and for a year or so (what felt like a lifetime to me back then) I had big red circles around my eyes and my mouth. I used to look in the mirror and think I looked like a clown. With four teeth removed during a minor operation, big metal braces (and lots more trauma with that experience for good measure) it wasn't my easiest few years, and certainly seemed to add to the increasing sense of discomfort I felt about what I looked like.

Around that time, I was also experiencing chronic pain in the form of headaches which were increasing in frequency. Over the following few years, this pain developed into something that was with me daily. Later in my teens, I started to experience long bouts of tiredness, and what I suspected at the time was correct, though it took 20 years to receive a formal diagnosis. I had developed the symptoms of ME, or myalgic encephalomyelitis, often referred to as chronic fatigue syndrome. The combination of these health challenges, and the all-consuming focus on trying to find treatments that might help me to get better, meant my BDD symptoms were dropped off the list as something that needed exploration or attention. They simply weren't shouting the loudest.

I needed some time out from the intensive dance training and so returned to the previous school I had attended, and it was there, during my A-levels, that I had my first significant introduction to Eastern philosophies. A woman from the Brahma Kumaris, a tradition loosely based on ancient Indian teachings, came to speak to us, and I went on to enjoy an introductory course they ran at the school. I immediately felt comfortable and at home with the basic concepts: there is something much bigger than what they called our 'little i'. This was the idea that we are much more than our job titles, roles, the stuff we own etc. I started to explore different types of meditation and continued to study with the Brahma Kumaris for a few years.

Then, in my early 20s, I found myself on a yoga teacher training course, something I did initially just for my own interest. I feel very blessed that I was guided to a diploma based on a type of yoga that is focused on a very individualised approach, the fundamentals of which I still benefit from today. The style I trained in is called viniyoga, which can be loosely translated as 'for the individual' (from Sanskrit, the prefixes denote the words 'adaptation', or 'appropriate application'). At that time, this focus was new to me. I was more familiar with the idea that yoga is predominantly a physical practice, with the philosophical aspects being merely a side benefit. Sadly, I think this view of yoga is all too common in the Western world, reinforced by our social media and Photoshop culture, which can often idolise youth and unrealistic body types.

Yoga and breathwork are some of the tools I can say with certainty have helped me to manage the BDD tendencies I experience and allow for a bigger perspective: a 'zooming out', if you will. I don't achieve this all the time, but in our imperfect, messy humanness, perhaps that's not achievable anyway. Something I learnt on my yoga course that stayed with me, and tied into earlier teachings I had come across, is the idea that we view the world through our own lens or, to use an analogy, through a pair of glasses. I remember making a drawing in my notes of a human head and an object, with a glass lens in between them that can get full of stuff. The memory of this drawing sticks with me for its simplicity and depth. I am sure many of you will already be familiar with this concept: the idea that throughout our childhood we experience many traumas and difficulties that gradually, over time, begin to colour the lens through which we see the world. It reminds me of a quote often attributed to Anaïs Nin: 'We don't see things as they are, we see them as we are.'

So, perhaps many of us would benefit from putting the difficult and complicated yoga postures to one side. The practice of yoga is, in my view, about gradually cleaning the lens so that we are more able to see things as they really are. Surely, no one ever achieves a perfectly clean lens. However, something I like to keep in mind when it comes to my physical and emotional recovery, and I think also applies here, is that it's about 'the overall direction of travel'. Or, as many yogis across time have expressed in their various ways, yoga is not about tying oneself up in knots, but rather undoing them.

When I remember to do so, I like to place my BDD thoughts inside that lens. One way I do that is to bring my awareness to the physical sensations in my body, the sounds and smells around me, or simply to my breath. I use the idea of returning to the present moment, a sense of coming home if you will. We see, in fact, this focus clearly laid out in the very fundamentals of yoga. If we go back to one of its principal ancient texts, the Yoga Sutras, a collection of Sanskrit sutras on the theory and practice of yoga, we read that yoga is 'the reducing of the fluctuations of the mind' (*yogaś-citta-vṛtti-nirodha*).

Another method I use to create some space between the stressful BBD thoughts and everything else is the concept of observation. In my yoga classes, I like to share the analogy that our thoughts are like clouds; they come and go, always changing and shifting. We can get very wrapped up in them, or we can have an awareness that we aren't the clouds, but rather the sky, and then just watch them pass on by with curiosity, and perhaps even some kindness. I don't always remember to do these things in the heat of the moment, but when I do, I find these practices give me really useful tools in my BDD toolbox.

Breathwork is another technique I find extremely helpful, especially working with the exhalation. Never underestimate the power of simple breath awareness. In yoga, we learn about the four parts of the breath: the inhale, the pause after the inhale, the exhale and the pause after the exhale. You don't have to do complicated pranayāma (the term for breathwork in yoga), or get into the lotus posture, to benefit from breathing practices. Long pauses between breaths are unreachable for many, and it is unwise to attempt anything but very fleeting pauses (unless you are working with an experienced breathwork practitioner). But the majority of us can access simple practices that can bring about profound benefits.

Of the four parts of the breath mentioned above, I like to focus primarily on one – the phrase I often return to is 'Exhale is king'. A practice that has helped me countless times over the years is that of gradually lengthening the exhalation. This could simply be for a fraction of a second, perhaps building up to a few seconds if you can manage it. You can count the length of the breath in your head or support your client to do so, but you don't have to (and it is important to never strain the breath in any way). Lengthening the exhalation can help us move into our parasympathetic nervous system, sometimes called our 'rest and digest' response, thus inviting a sense of relaxation and energy-replenishment into the body.

Using breath awareness has been a really effective tool for me over the years to help bring myself more fully into my body and shift away from my 'monkey mind', the place where my BDD thoughts like to hang out. I often think of what a therapist said to me when I was having Somatic Experiencing sessions, a type of treatment that helps people to find healing from trauma. The practitioner said something along the lines of, 'It's not about never leaving your body; it's about noticing when you've gone, and knowing how to come back.' The breath can be a fantastic bridge back into awareness of our body.

I want to finish by sharing something that a support-group participant gifted us with during one of the wonderful online BDD and mindfulness groups I attend, a space that has been a huge support and comfort to me over the last three years. It's something that has stayed with me, and I return to it again and again. I will paraphrase what they said (shared with permission):

> It's not about curing. It's about, 'How can I hold it? How can I be a BDD ninja?' I'm less interested in getting well than I used to be. I can see your okayness and I can feel mine, and that's good enough for today.

Chapter 7

BDD and the Family

Using Principles of Non-Violent Resistance and Yoga
to Support Families with BDD in Their Midst

———

JILL LUBIENSKI

As a Family and Systemic Psychotherapist and Social Worker, my experience with families within which there is a family member experiencing body dysmorphic disorder (BDD) and associated struggles is that they are in need of professional support and guidance which attends to the needs of all those involved, and which recognises the multi-faceted nature of the causal factors underlying and perpetuating the BDD. The personal qualities in the practitioner are key to a successful outcome. In particular, it is necessary for practitioners to resist the temptation to apportion blame and, rather, to appreciate the importance of alliance building with parents, families and the systems around them as being key to raising each person's sense of agency, and in moving from a position of helplessness to action to support themselves and/or their loved one.

My focus is on practical approaches which offer guidance in what to do in situations of intense stress. This chapter is an attempt to offer some of my experience to others. I have developed an integrated approach which draws on my training as a Systemic Psychotherapist and as an accredited practitioner of Non-Violent Resistance Parent Therapy (NVR), a systemic intervention developed by Haim Omer and his clinical team in Tel Aviv, Israel (Omer, 2004, 2021). This applies the philosophy, principles and methods of non-violent resistance from the social and political sphere and the work of Mahatma Gandhi and Martin Luther King into the family domain. In addition to this, I have been practising yoga for over 35 years and am trained as a yoga teacher. I have been experimenting with integrating some yoga-based methods, working on the mind–body connection and on health promotion for those I work with. NVR is also essentially yoga, in its widest sense, which I will talk more about later in this chapter also.

NVR was developed to work directly with the parent or carer of a struggling child or young person, providing them with, as Haim Omer phrases it, 'a parental North' (Omer, 2021, p.2): a map which offers them a way out of a situation when they feel, as one parent said to me recently, 'like I'm in a fog and going round and round and getting nowhere'. It will be useful as a starting point, to provide a brief overview of NVR and its main principles and methods, including its application to the experience of BDD in particular.

NVR begins by highlighting, in discussion with the family, how the family respond to a person in times of stress, anger or violence and, importantly, how escalation happens at home, so this can be minimised. Often parents, for example, talk about 'walking on eggshells' with their child (or partner in the context of adult experiences of BDD), afraid to upset them due to fears of ever more dangerous levels of confrontation and gradually submitting to the increasing demands of the BDD in an attempt to keep the peace and avoid a crisis. If we think about this principle more broadly, we could also consider how people's experience may be of 'walking on eggshells' with their BDD – afraid, for example, not to repeatedly look into the mirror in case it provokes an increase of anxiety.

Symmetrical and Complementary Escalation

Ideas of symmetrical and complementary escalation (Patterson et al. 1984; Patterson, Reid & Dishion, 1992, both cited in Omer, 2021, p. 68) are utilised in NVR to delineate escalation processes. When a parent, partner or family as a whole continually submit to the demands of the BDD – becoming increasingly anxious and helpless while attempting to keep the peace to avoid causing or increasing upset, anger or aggression – they have entered into complementary escalation. You may have also heard of it referred to in other disciplines as 'family accommodation'. In the same way, by continually submitting to the demands of their BDD, a person can get locked into a cycle of submissiveness, restriction and increasing safety behaviours. This can set up a cycle of anxiety and avoidance which perpetuates the person's and family members' distress and sense of being unable to find a way forward or to cope.

NVR helps families to recognise how escalation happens in their home and to focus on their responses and reactions: to quote Gandhi, to 'be the change they wish to see in the world'. This gradually changes the environment around the person and moves family members away from the extremes of permissive and/or authoritarian styles without themselves becoming violent or escalating conflict.

Parental Presence

Haim Omer developed the concept of 'parental presence' as being central to the aims of NVR: this can also be applied with other family members, for example 'partner presence' or 'sibling presence' for and with the person experiencing BDD. Parental presence is developed in three main contexts: internally in the *embodied* presence of the parent who is coached and supported to develop self-control to avoid escalation by walking away and deferring their response; *physically* in the way the parent is encouraged to stay in the spaces inhabited by the child; and *systemically* by breaking the veil of secrecy surrounding the situation at home, and requesting and utilising specific types of support from other adults. Again, each of these principles can also be applied to the internal experience of BDD, i.e. through developing agency over BDD-related behaviours; to face rather than avoid BDD; and by requesting support from others including family, friends and, where desired and appropriate, mental health professionals.

The Announcement

From discussions around escalation processes, the importance of de-escalation and the central concept of developing parental presence, the active protest methods are introduced. These are: *the Announcement, Recruiting Supporters, the Sit In* and *Reconciliation Gestures*, as well as other methods for increasing parental/partner/sibling etc. presence. The Announcement is a one-off ritual wherein the parent/partner delivers a written statement to the person in which they are clear about resisting the BDD and associated behaviours and struggles non-violently; that they will no longer stay alone in trying to deal with the situation; that they will be getting help from other trusted adults; and that they love the person and want to reclaim their lives and future as a family together. The Announcement is a written commitment spoken aloud in a calm, measured manner and which symbolises a turning point in how they intend to go forwards. The NVR practitioner supporting the family carefully plans and prepares the delivery and timing of the Announcement with the family member or members, preparing them for possible emotional and resistant reactions. In the same way, an Announcement could be written and read by supporters such as family members or friends of an adult experiencing BDD; or the person experiencing BDD themselves might write such an Announcement and share it with supportive others as a way of 'drawing a line in the sand' with their BDD.

An Announcement made by the parents to their teenager experiencing BDD may look something like this:

> Jenny, we love you so much. We see how caring and sensitive you are with animals and with your young cousins, and what a talent you have for drawing. We also know that life has been so hard for you recently, as BDD tells you that you appear ugly and unacceptable to others and increases feelings of anxiety and depression, so you feel the need to repeatedly check yourself in the mirror and ask us constantly for reassurance. Often you become upset and angry with us when we do not immediately do the things you need us to do to keep BDD quiet. This is interfering with your life, and your education, friendships and hobbies. It is also affecting our relationship with you, as we argue so much and you no longer wish to spend time with us and your brother. We worry about how alone you are.

> We realise it is very hard to ignore BDD. We see how distressed you are in trying to cope with your fears. We are also aware that our behaviour so far has not helped you. We have tried to provide you with the reassurance you seek and have at times become angry and frustrated that you do not believe us. We have also sometimes tried to ignore BDD and made demands that you do the same, which we see now has not been helpful. We realise that if you could simply ignore BDD, you would, and we do not blame you for any of this.

> We are now getting some help for ourselves, as we are your parents and it is our job to help you with your suffering. We understand more about BDD than we did before, and we will do our best to help you to trust us, so we can help you to not give into BDD. We have made a decision that we need to do a better job of helping you to overcome this.

> We will, therefore, no longer try to cope with this alone. We will be getting help from friends, family and professionals who we believe can support us all. We will give you as much help as we can to resist the distressing

effects BDD has on you and on those who love you; this could include agreeing to therapy for yourself, if you want it.

We will be talking with you some more about our ideas to support you. We cannot do this alone – but together we are strong! We look forward to the future with hope, remembering the happy times we spent as a family in the past. You are our sensitive, kind and funny daughter who possesses such wisdom, wit and humour and who has brought so much fun and laughter into our home.

With love

Mum and Dad

Recruiting Supporters

In writing and delivering an Announcement, the family member or members are committing to Recruiting Supporters. The NVR practitioner coaches the family member(s) in this task, helping them to resist default positions of emphasising the need to maintain privacy and, instead, centring their own immediate needs for support, working to develop a wide network of support over time. This is a central condition for the success of NVR, as it helps to reduce a family's sense of isolation and separateness by talking to others and thereby acquiring specific and targeted help. Supporters are also crucial for helping family members and/or people with lived experience of BDD in their acts of peaceful presence-raising and resistance against any harmful and self-destructive behaviours. Supporters assist with Announcements and with Sit Ins also.

Sit Ins

Sit Ins are carefully planned presence-raising acts following a harmful act, where a family member or members come closer to the person and sit with them to let them know they are resisting, for example, the safety behaviours related to the BDD and would like the person to think of a different way forward. Sit Ins utilise three important principles: time, closeness and silence. They are time-limited, usually taking place in the person's bedroom or similar. They can last for up to an hour when a family member is skilled enough to withstand any pressures and protests from the person by remaining silent and not escalating or becoming distressed. Coaching, detailed planning, preparation and role-play all assist the family member in building their non-violent resistance skills in the face of continued upset and any provocation or demands, such as for cosmetic surgery. When choosing the best time for a Sit In, it is helpful to consider Haim Omer's suggestion to 'strike when the iron is cold'.

Reconciliation Gestures

Threaded through these presence-raising acts are Reconciliation Gestures: caring, connective acts designed to promote the sense that the family members can remain connected to their loved one even in the face of the pain and struggle of BDD. The family member(s) can offer care, love and concern to a person even during strong BDD behaviours and 'episodes'. This strengthens the image of the family member(s) as loving in the mind of the person while reducing any sense of demonisation. One parent bought a T shirt with the message 'You cannot divorce me!' printed on the front as a way of symbolising this ongoing struggle to reclaim their role as the parent who loves, guides and supports their child – a parent who, in other words, displays parental presence in all the forms I mentioned earlier.

New Applications of NVR

Over the years since 2004, when Haim Omer published his first book on NVR outlining the methods and approach detailed earlier in this chapter, many new applications of the approach have grown. Notable developments include work on multi-stressed families by Jakob (2018, 2019) which includes developing a safe support network, addressing trauma – including transgenerational trauma – and enlivening the caring dialogue between parent and child. Other adaptations include treating childhood anxiety disorders (Leibowitz & Omer, 2013) and adult entrenched dependency (Dulberger & Omer, 2021). The application of NVR and anxiety disorders is particularly relevant and useful in terms of assisting families experiencing BDD. Leibowitz and Omer (2013, pp. 157–233) have developed a model of NVR which combines NVR and CBT (Cognitive Behavioural Therapy) called Supportive Parenting for Anxious Childhood Emotions (SPACE). This approach acknowledges that there is often literally a loss of mental and physical space for parents in situations where they are living with a highly anxious and distressed child, such as in the case of BDD; and the same can be said for living with a partner experiencing BDD also. SPACE aims to restore family structure, routine and overall family functioning in a way which enhances each person's ability to regulate themselves and which contains the person experiencing the BDD.

The SPACE model is focused very specifically on the areas of developing a supportive position, reducing potential for escalation and disharmony between family members, and uniting them to validate the person's fears as legitimate, alongside a message of belief in the person's ability to cope in a targeted and goal-based manner. Parental/partner accommodation is also focused on, with the therapist helping parents/partners to delineate how they accommodate or assist the person's BDD. These include participating in rituals such as obsessive body checking; answering questions related to BDD concerns; preparing and purchasing particular items of clothing designed to conceal the body area of concern; not inviting guests into the house; accompanying the person for unnecessary medical check-ups or consultations related to changing a body part; and helping to research costly and unnecessary cosmetic procedures.

SPACE treatment is focused on supporting the family member to remain in a caring position without over-protecting, over-demanding or perpetuating overreliance. The goal is to help the person develop anxiety regulation strategies and to become more self-reliant. As part of the intervention, and particularly where heightened emotions and resistance from the person are predicted, the NVR methods discussed earlier may be introduced. An example would be the delivery of an Announcement to inform the person of the family members' intention to act without being drawn into escalatory interactions, and to begin the process of focusing on their own actions and reactions rather than trying to change the person. A person may also be told about any intentions to involve supporters which will strengthen their resolve and likely help them to stay in a place of non-violence and non-escalation.

The SPACE model is also one which emphasises other key developments in NVR, such as the concepts of New Authority (Omer, 2011) and the Parental Anchoring Function (Omer, Satran & Dritter, 2017). New Authority offers a model of relationship based on family members being emotionally closer to the person; being obviously present in the life and the mind of the person; exercising and modelling self-control and personal responsibility; asking for and accepting support; and persevering and persisting in the face of difficulties rather than insisting on immediate and arbitrary compliance. This is a model, perhaps, which feels acceptable in a 21st century society, which increasingly rejects authoritarian attitudes and distance while simultaneously understanding that parents and other family members have a key role in offering safety, security, guidance and wisdom.

The concept of the Parental Anchoring Function is a symbol of attachment and of each person's need for security and safety. This symbol can offer guidance to family members who feel they are being engulfed by the tidal waves of BDD, including through experiencing fears for themselves and their loved one. NVR adapted via the SPACE model is a way for family members to attain an anchored position.

In working directly with families in this way, I have noticed how much they benefit from techniques to manage their own high arousal levels and find their own internal anchors before taking the action they have committed to in the NVR/SPACE frame. As part of this process, I utilise yoga breathwork techniques (pranayama) along with easy-to-learn yoga postures (asanas).

The Place of Yoga within the NVR Approach

There are many ways of defining 'yoga', for example to 'come together' or 'to unite'. Another meaning is 'to attain what was previously unattainable... In fact, every change is yoga' (Desikachar, 1995, pp. 5, 6). There are also many ways of practising yoga. In the West, we often tend to think of yoga as just the physical poses or asanas, though there are also the practices of meditation, breathing and of studying the yoga sutras of Patanjali – teachings which are often seen as the heart of yoga.

Sutras are short and distilled teachings, universal to humankind, which give the means for self-understanding. We can think of yoga as a vehicle for gaining self-understanding through the Yamas and Niyamas. Broadly speaking, these are ethical instructions of what not to do and what do, respectively. The Yamas and Niyamas focus on our attitudes and behaviours towards ourselves and others and are the first two of what we know as the eight limbs of yoga. Patanjali's Yoga Sutras mentions five Yamas, the first of which is Ahimsa. Ahimsa is often thought to mean non-violence; however, in its widest sense, it means behaving with kindness and consideration for others. Gandhi adopted the study of the Yamas in his life, calling his autobiography *The Story of My Experiments with Truth* (1925), which relates specifically to the Yama of Brahmacarya, or 'the movement towards the essential...it means responsible behaviour with respect to our goal of moving toward the truth' (Desikachar, 1995, p. 99). Gandhi practised Ahimsa and the other Yamas in a pure form and lived his life in his later years in a very spiritually focused manner, which is not compatible with the life of most ordinary citizens. However, we can all adopt consideration of the Yamas in guiding us on a path of pondering and actioning how we relate to others and to ourselves.

My personal practice of NVR as an intervention aligns with my philosophy and view of the world as a yoga practitioner in the widest sense. There is no requirement for a family member or therapist to adopt such a position, but for me it allows an authenticity to infuse my practice, alongside using the methods with as much integrity as I can in a self-reflexive way. I view my journey as a practitioner as paralleling the family's journeys in terms of increasing self-knowledge and understanding. I practise Ahimsa in my way of being with families, inviting them to co-create the intervention, and offering an attitude of respect for their resilience and commitment to their family in the face of great challenges. When I introduce a yoga breathing technique or asana to parents or loved ones as part of NVR, I do so from a position of not being insistent or convinced of the rightness of my way of doing things, but as an offering of something which may support them in walking an increasingly balanced and peaceful path with their loved one.

I will detail a few yoga exercises here which can be used by practitioners to stabilise themselves before sessions, and for the practitioner to teach family members to use at any time they may need them, for example for self-regulation. Personally, I have found yoga so helpful in this way within my therapeutic practice.

When my work context allows, before a session with a family, I like to sit quietly, connect my awareness to my body sitting in the chair and take a few seconds to do a body scan from head to toe, bringing my awareness to my breath and relaxing each part of the body in turn. If time allows, at this point I may practise one of the pranayama exercises detailed here. A favourite of mine for its soothing effects is Nadi Shodhana (alternate nostril breathing). I then mentally 'tune in' to the family I am seeing, connecting to them before we meet in person, and imagining what their concerns are and what I need to do to open myself to understanding each of them. I focus particularly on connecting mind and heart as I wish to offer a balance of compassion, kindness and empathy alongside my knowledge and skills as a therapist. If I bring in all parts of myself, steady my mind and body, and learn to respond rather than react, I can offer a creative approach in situations of high stress, rather than becoming caught up in the anxiety threatening to engulf the family.

Bhramari Breath: Bumble Bee Breath

This breathing technique relaxes the autonomic nervous system and balances emotional and mental states as it calms overwhelming thoughts. When we lengthen the exhale to be longer than the inhale we activate the parasympathetic nervous system, the energising-conserving, rest-and-digest part of our nervous system, thus igniting the relaxation response.

Do not force the breath. Take it gently, yet the longer the buzzing exhalation, the more relaxing tends to be the effect.

- Sit in a comfortable position with a long spine and relax the shoulders and neck.

- Inhale and exhale in a natural way a few times.

- Close the mouth and lips, placing the tongue towards the back of the top teeth.

- Place the forefingers in the ears if it feels comfortable for you to do so.

- Breathe in deeply.

- Exhale and make a buzzing sound in the throat, like a bee.

- Feel the vibration in the skull and head.

- Repeat by inhaling through the nose and exhale humming like a bee.

Listening to the buzzing draws the senses inwards and calms a busy mind.

Nadi Shodhana: Alternate Nostril Breathing

This pranayama exercise opens both nostrils and stimulates the left and right hemispheres of the brain, balancing brain activity. It also lowers the heart rate and reduces stress. It is sometimes called 'neuro-respiratory breathing' (Chopra, 2001, pp. 358–359). By increasing the regularity of the breath, the entire nervous system is soothed. Again, as with all the exercises, it is important not to strain.

- Find a quiet place.

- Do not hold the breath, and there is no need to count the inhale and exhale.

- Sit in a comfortable position with a long spine and relax the shoulders and neck.

- Gently close the right nostril with the thumb.

- Slowly exhale through the left nostril.

- Inhale through the left nostril.

- Close the left nostril with the middle two fingers and open the right nostril.

- Exhale through the right nostril.

- Inhale through the right nostril.

- The breath should be easy, smooth and steady, not forced.

- Continue for up to five minutes, morning and evening.

Wide-Legged Camel Forward Fold (seated)

Avoid if you have a back injury.

This can be done at a desk or in a chair. It counteracts any hunching of the chest and shoulders. As it is a forward fold, it can release spinal tension and calm the mind.

- Sit forward on the front of the chair and take the feet wide.

- Inhale, sweeping the arms overhead.

- Exhale, placing the hands to the bottom of the chair back.

- Inhale and lift the chest upwards and hold for a count of five or whatever feels comfortable.

- Clasp the hands behind the back.

- Exhale and fold forward, lifting the arms gently and pressing the feet into the floor.

- Hold for a count of five, or whatever feels comfortable, then release the hands and come up slowly.

Tadasana: Mountain Pose

This basic posture brings awareness of the body, especially of the spine, and promotes the experience of stillness, strength, stability and centring. As Maharishi Mahesh Yogi (Founder of the Transcendental Meditation Movement) said, 'If we are strong and stable, we can set our sail with any wind that comes along. We make up our own direction.'

This posture may help parents to imagine themselves as securely anchored against the waves of their child's anxiety which is threatening to unmoor them.

- Distribute the weight evenly on the feet.

- Engage the thighs to lift the kneecaps slightly.

- Pull in the lower belly.

- Lengthen through the spine, tucking in the chin slightly.

- Lengthen the sides of the body.

- Lift the chest.

- Broaden the collarbones.

- Relax the shoulders.

- Release any tension in the hands.

- Relax the jaw.

- Soften the forehead.

Feel the dual qualities of softness and strength and the flow of energy within. Notice what you are holding on to and what you can let go of.

Virabhadrasana: Warrior Two

Virabhadra was a warrior from Hindu mythology, so you could think of this pose as activating your inner warrior, cultivating willpower, energy and focus, and amplifying your determination to resist the distressing effects of BDD in the family.

- Start in Tadasana as described earlier.

- Take a wide stance, about a leg length.

- Keeping the left foot facing the long length of your mat, turn the right foot towards the short edge of your mat. You can align the heel of the right foot with the arch of the left foot if you like.

- Connect your feet fully to the mat.

- Extend your arms and raise them to shoulder height.

- Bend the right knee, placing it directly above the right ankle.

- Sink the hips down.

- Look towards the middle finger of the outstretched right hand.

- Relax the shoulders, open the chest.

- Breathe naturally and hold for as long as is comfortable.

- To come out, straighten your right leg and turn your feet parallel again.

- Repeat on the left side.

I encourage parents I work with to also teach these methods of self-regulation to their child or young person. It is typically helpful for children to see their parents or carers working on their own arousal levels and taking responsibility for these to reduce escalation and bring more containment to themselves and their relationships.

Concluding Reflections

Family members often disconnect and lose their presence in order to survive in very difficult and prolonged situations of stress and distress, such as within the context of a loved one experiencing BDD. If experiences of trauma are left unaddressed, escalation is likely to continue and to further embed destructive communication patterns. NVR involves careful listening to each family member to hear about their particular experience and how they have been affected. It is a privilege to witness how family members recover something of themselves as the focus is placed on their needs while their suffering is acknowledged and worked with directly.

NVR gives both family members and practitioners practical methods and allows for their creativity and resourcefulness to enable more peaceful, calm and harmonious family relationships. Once escalation, aggression, and safety behaviours have diminished, the needs of the person experiencing BDD can be perceived more clearly and addressed more appropriately and effectively.

References

Chopra, D. (2001). *Perfect health: The complete mind body guide*, Revised edn. Bantam Books.

Desikachar, T. K. V. (1995). *The heart of yoga: Developing a personal practice*. Inner Traditions International.

Dulberger, D., & Omer, H. (2021). *Non-emerging adulthood: Helping the parents of adult children with entrenched dependence*. Cambridge University Press.

Jakob, P. (2018). Multi-stressed families, child violence and the larger system: An adaptation of the non-violent model. *Journal of Family Therapy, 40*, 25–44.

Jakob, P. (2019). Child-focussed family therapy using non-violent resistance: Hearing the voice of need in the traumatized child. In E. Heismann, J. Jude & E. Day (eds), *Non-violent resistance: Innovations in practice* (pp. 51–63). Pavilion Publishing and Media.

Leibowitz, E., & Omer, H. (2013). *Treating childhood and adolescent anxiety: A guide for caregivers*. Wiley.

Omer, H. (2004). *Non-violent resistance: A new approach to violent and self-destructive children*. Cambridge University Press.

Omer, H. (2011). *The new authority: Family, school and community*. Cambridge University Press.

Omer, H. (2021). *Non-violent resistance: A new approach to violent and self destructive children*, 2nd edn. Cambridge University Press.

Omer, H., Satran, S., & Dritter, O. (2017). Vigilant care: An integrative reformulation regarding parental monitoring. *Psychological Review, 123*, 291–304.

Chapter 8

The Autonomic Nervous System and the Window of Tolerance in BDD

———

NICOLE SCHNACKENBERG

This chapter offers a broad-brush overview of the autonomic nervous system and some of the potential implications this understanding may have for the experience of body dysmorphic disorder (BDD). It also considers some simple ways of supporting the nervous system to come into balance and of increasing the 'Window of Tolerance': a concept we will explore later in the chapter.

The autonomic nervous system is the part of the nervous system which supplies the internal organs, including the blood vessels, stomach, intestine, kidney, liver, bladder, genitals, pupils, heart and sweat, salivary and digestive glands. It regulates certain body processes such as breathing rate, heart rate and digestion. This system operates autonomously, without conscious effort.

There are two main branches or divisions of the autonomic nervous system: the sympathetic (energy mobilising) branch and the parasympathetic (energy conserving) branch. The majority of the ganglia (structures containing nerve cell bodies) for the sympathetic nervous system are located on either side of the spinal cord, just outside of it. The ganglia for the parasympathetic nervous system are located near or in the organs they connect with.

It is not the case that one branch of the autonomic nervous system is 'switched on' at any one time while the other is 'switched off'. We can think of the system as operating more like a dimmer switch than a light switch, with both branches operational at any one time, yet one can be more active than the other. Depending on aspects of one's developmental and medical histories, and on life experiences, a person might have a propensity to be more sympathetically or parasympathetically dominated. Likewise, there may be times of the day, week, month etc. and certain experiences throughout the day and in the course of the lifespan that activate one branch more strongly than the other.

When the sympathetic nervous system is dominant, the:

- heart rate increases

- blood pressure increases

- body temperature increases

- pupils dilate

- blood rushes to the extremities.

Conversely, when the parasympathetic nervous system dominates:

- heart rate decreases

- blood pressure decreases

- body temperature decreases

- pupils contract

- blood rushes to the visceral organs.

The sympathetic nervous system is sometimes colloquially referred to as the 'fight, flight, freeze, fawn' branch of the autonomic nervous system and the parasympathetic branch as the 'rest and digest' division. However, it is important to note that, when balanced, the sympathetic nervous system mobilises the body to get out of bed in the morning, to talk, to eat, to move etc., and only tips into a fight/flight/freeze/fawn state when it becomes hyper-aroused. The parasympathetic branch on the other hand, when in balance, facilitates times of rest and the ability to fall asleep at night, among numerous other functions.

The Window of Tolerance and Polyvagal Theory

When the sympathetic branch of the autonomic nervous system becomes strongly aroused, igniting sensations like a racing heart, tingling arms and legs, a fast and shallow breathing rate etc., the person has entered an anxiety response. Conversely, when the parasympathetic branch becomes acutely active, a person may enter a numb, depressed and even dissociated state. Between these states of hyper-arousal and hypo-arousal sits the Window of Tolerance (Siegel, 1999): a space within which one can think and feel at the same time; have a sense of being safe and connected to others; and believe in one's ability to cope and maintain a semblance of self-efficacy emotionally.

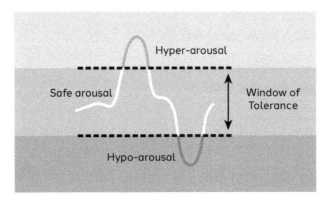

WINDOW OF TOLERANCE

As I have written about elsewhere (Schnackenberg, 2019), the psycho-biology of shame, including in relation to the Window of Tolerance, is particularly pertinent when considering the experience of BDD. In early episodes of shame, the infant encounters looking at the primary caregiver 'like smiling at a stranger' (Tomkins, 1963, p. 123). Expecting an exchange of psycho-biologically attuned, shared positive affect, the infant instead experiences a facially expressed misattunement, triggering a shock-induced deflation (Schore, 2002). The infant is, thus, propelled into a low-arousal state they cannot yet autoregulate. Therefore, shame represents a rapid transition from a pre-existing, high-arousal, positive state to a low-arousal, negative state (a decrescendo (Stern, 1985)). Physiologically, this represents a shift from sympathetic to parasympathetic predominant activity, induced through vagal activity (a dorsal vagal response (Porges, 1995; Schore, 1998)). With this comes the slowing of the heart rate, and the sense of time slowing down, which may magnify anything occurring during the state of shame. Given that shame has been described as a largely visual experience, it is perhaps unsurprising that, for some people (including in the context of BDD), it is the visual aspects of the self and their perceived appearance to another that become magnified.

The Window of Tolerance model relates to the three lines of defence outlined in Polyvagal Theory (Porges, 2011). Essentially, when humans experience a felt sense of danger (either externally or internally, for example in the form of unsettling or even frightening bodily sensations and thoughts) the first thing we tend to do is to attempt to socially engage: we try to bring people close and to receive comfort from them. It is important to note, however, that if a person has had difficult or even traumatic relational experiences in the past or is afraid of people seeing, touching and judging them in the present (as is typically the case with BDD), or indeed if there is nobody around to connect with and from whom to seek soothing, a person may 'skip' this step and go straight to the second line of defence: heightened sympathetic nervous system arousal (depicted in the model as above the Window of Tolerance).

Within the second line of defence, humans attempt to run away or avoid the perceived danger. In the context of BDD this may mean fleeing social groups, covering up or avoiding mirrors, or escaping into safety behaviours. One may also attempt to fight, perhaps lashing out at others or oneself (for example in the form of skin picking, which incidentally can also be conceptualised as a flight response). Additionally, a person may go into freeze mode or begin to fawn – to lay aside their needs servilely to keep another pacified (and this 'other' could be the BDD) .

If the person is unable to escape or fight back in any way, or feels these actions will not serve to keep them safe, they may come to the (conscious, semi-conscious or unconscious) realisation that the dreaded thing, whatever that may be, is going to happen. In the context of BDD, this could be a felt sense that they are going to be mocked or ridiculed, or that an internal disgust reaction to the perceived defect is going to occur, and that nothing can be done to remove oneself from the situation or thwart this perceived reaction. Thus, the person may go into the third line of defence: dorsal vagal system activation, which is a parasympathetic response. In this state, the person disconnects from the interoceptive signals of the body and there is a dissociation from emotion. This is both a protective and adaptive response: to become numb and enter into a dissociated state so as not to feel the terrifying sensations and emotions arising in the body.

In the following figure, Polyvagal Theory is embedded into the Window of Tolerance model.

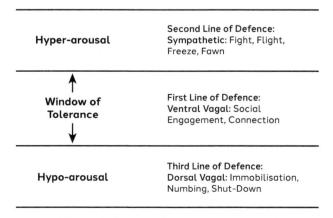

WINDOW OF TOLERANCE AND POLYVAGAL MODEL
Adapted from Ogden, Minton & Pain (2006, pp. 27, 32); Corrigan, Fisher & Nutt (2011, p. 2)

Depending on developmental history and life experiences, some people may sometimes, or even regularly, go straight into the third line of defence when they experience those initial body-based sensations related to a felt sense of unsafety and fear. They may rapidly dissociate from sensations and emotions and find themselves regularly in a highly numb and disconnected state. The propensity to go directly to the second or third line of defence can also be a ramification of developmental trauma (see Chapter 2 for Arie Winograd's description of such trauma and its array of possible implications in the context of BDD).

In the context of BDD, the safety behaviours can become the 'go to' strategy used to bring oneself back into the Window of Tolerance, understandably and adaptively so. The difficulty with this is that while engagement in safety behaviours may alleviate the felt sense anxiety or lift the mood in the short term, engaging in safety behaviours like mirror checking or mirror avoidance is very unlikely to make a person feel better in the long term, or do anything to expand the Window of Tolerance overall. Furthermore, escaping into safety behaviours can stimulate and perpetuate a self-amplifying cycle; in other words, a cycle of more and more safety behaviours or an increasing number of repetitions of the safety behaviours. This is partially because the nervous system tends to habituate to stimuli; thus, touching the skin to check for blemishes once every hour, for example, might initially be enough to soothe the anxiety and calm the sympathetic branch of the autonomic nervous system. But later, as the nervous system recalibrates to this checking, the person may need to check more and more often, and for longer and longer periods, to produce the same calming and soothing effect.

Experimenting with replacing safety behaviours with other mechanisms for coming into the Window of Tolerance may, therefore, be considerably more supportive and beneficial in the long term than the short-term soothing brought about by the safety behaviours. Below are some ideas, although it is important to note that the nervous system of each human being is nuanced and unique. It is recommended to support your client in drawing up their own table, considering the activities, foods, scents etc. which calm them down and those which pep them up. The ideas below, nevertheless, may be a helpful starting point.

Soothing (during times of anxiety) Activates the parasympathetic (energy conserving) branch of the autonomic nervous system	Energising (during times of low mood) Activates the sympathetic (energy mobilising) branch of the autonomic nervous system
Low, slow breathing with extended exhalations, e.g. breathing in for the count of three and out for the count of six	Breathing with extended inhalations, e.g. breathing in for the count of six and out for the count of three
Breathing in and out through the left nostril while lightly blocking the right nostril	Breathing in and out through the right nostril while lightly blocking the left nostril
Slow swaying, rocking, swinging	Jogging, skipping, trampolining
Gentle, repetitive yoga, Tai Chi, Qi Gong etc.	Faster-paced yoga, dance etc.
Gentle music with a repetitive rhythm	Upbeat, pacy music
Chamomile tea	Ginger tea
Root vegetables, porridge oats	Tropical fruits
Dimmed lighting	Bright lighting
Warm bath	Cold or cool shower

Some clients I have worked with have found it helpful to have a copy of their table in their pockets, ready to pull out and consult for alternatives when intrusive thoughts and accompanying compulsions arise.

In terms of expanding the Window of Tolerance more generally, the following pointers may be helpful.

Experiment with:

- Reducing or eliminating caffeine, including in beverages like cola and food items like chocolate (caffeine is sympathetically arousing, taxing to the nervous system and can reduce the 'bandwidth' of the Window of Tolerance).

- Increasing intake of Omega-3 fatty acids and green vegetables.

- Improving sleep patterns, prioritising at least some sleep between the hours of 10 pm and midnight if possible.

- Stimulating the vagus nerve (integral to Polyvagal Theory and the three lines of defence) daily to improve vagal tone through singing, humming and gargling.

- Regular engagement in breath-led movement practices like yoga or Tai Chi.

- Cold or cool showers; cool water swimming.

Many of the Polyvagal-Theory exercises and tools offered by clinician Deb Dana (2018, 2020, 2021) can also be usefully employed with working with people experiencing BDD, including mapping the nervous system (Dana, 2018), and identifying *ventral vagal anchors* (Dana, 2020), which are the experiences that help a person to anchor in the ventral vagal state using the categories of *who, what, where* and *when*. When using these tools with clients experiencing BDD, it is important to remember that the first line of defence – connection – may have itself become frightening due to past experiences of relational trauma and an intense fear of rejection. Thus, gentleness, openness, patience and curiosity are essential within the process.

Heart-Rate Variability

The phenomenon of heart rate variability is an important consideration when thinking about expanding the Window of Tolerance. Heart rate variability, or HRV, is the variance in time between the beats of the heart, controlled by the autonomic nervous system. When one is in a state of sympathetic nervous system hyper-arousal, the HRV is low; there is less variance in the intervals between each heartbeat. In a more relaxed state, i.e. when one is within their Window of Tolerance, the variability is higher.

The more flexible the autonomic nervous system is to both responding to and re-regulating after arousing/frightening experiences in the environment, the wider the Window of Tolerance is and becomes. Low HRV is associated with worsening experiences of both depression and anxiety and is correlated with an increased risk of cardiovascular disease. Therefore, improving one's HRV and, thus, expanding the Window of Tolerance has important implications for both physical and emotional health.

There are some electronic applications (apps) accompanied with inexpensive heart rate monitors available for exploring HRV. One such app I use regularly with clients and personally to pleasing effect is a piece of biofeedback software called emWave by HeartMath. EmWave measures HRV in real time via a simple ear-clip. It also comes with various mindfulness tools and games. As the HRV increases through the application of breathing practices, for example, a hot air balloon begins to fly through the sky on the screen. Thus, one can practise increasing their HRV and Window of Tolerance. Seeing this happen in real time on the screen can make it easier to internalise and therefore use the experience of self-regulation in other situations and contexts.

Regulating the Nervous System

It can be supportive to encourage your client to keep a reflective journal about how the actions they are exploring (in an attempt to regulate the nervous system and expand the Window of Tolerance) are affecting and working for them, updating the table/list of up- and down-regulators as necessary and amending the practices to best suit and support them. It is vital to remind your client not to lose hope if some things do not seem to be having the desired effect. Support your client to take on the role of an investigator and to continue to try out different possibilities until they find something that works effectively for them. Sometimes it is helpful to consider these practices in light of the safety behaviours a person may have typically gone to in the past. For example, if your client tends to pick their skin when they are feeling anxious it might be helpful to support them to think about something they could do with that same body part, i.e. the fingers, to bring themselves back into their Window of Tolerance, such as knitting, weaving, drawing/painting, sculpting, weeding, unpicking stitches on a seam etc.

Clients may also find it helpful to be reminded to take care of and be gentle with themselves after intense times of sympathetic hyper-arousal.

After a period of intense anxiety, the nervous system tends to 'crash' down into a parasympathetic state. Clients might find themselves feeling acutely exhausted and as though they cannot focus on work, feel moved to withdraw from others for a while etc. Self-care is vital at these times. Taking a nap may be the kindest course of action, or perhaps a warm bath or some time alone with a relaxing hobby or listening to calming music. This might include letting others who are worried about the person (and may have been present during the anxiety-state) know that they are 'coming down' from feeling hyper-aroused and now need to rest a little in order to feel restored and ready to talk, continue with their day in the way they had previously planned and so on.

It can be extremely beneficial, thus, to allow one's nervous system the recuperation time it needs. Chamomile or lavender tea may be supportive at this time, as may a warm blanket wrapped fairly tightly around the person and time to be alone or next to a quiet, containing other (i.e. person or pet), depending on what helps each person the most. It can be helpful to support your client to draw up a list of soothing practices they can go to after times of sympathetic hyper-arousal/anxiety/distress.

Breathing Practices for Nervous System Regulation

In the first part of this chapter, we explored some of the nuances of the autonomic nervous system and considered potential ways both of expanding the Window of Tolerance and of soothing states of hypo- and hyper-arousal. In the second half of this chapter, we will focus on breathing techniques and practices specifically.

Each time we take an in-breath (an inhalation) the sympathetic (energy mobilising) branch of the autonomic nervous system is activated. And each time we exhale, we stimulate the parasympathetic (energy conserving) branch. Therefore, one of the simplest things one can do to activate either branch of the autonomic nervous system is to lengthen the inhalation or the exhalation (ideally for at least 10–12 rounds).

It can be helpful to let your client know that lengthening the inhalation, making it longer than the exhalation, will stimulate the sympathetic (energy mobilising branch) of the autonomic nervous system, thus helping to bring themselves 'up' into their Window of Tolerance from states of numbness and depression. Conversely, they can make the exhalation longer than the inhalation to stimulate the parasympathetic (energy conserving) branch and bring themselves down from states of anxiety and hyper-arousal. I recommend experimenting with your client with different time intervals to find their 'sweet spot', i.e. gradually lengthening the exhalation to a place which feels both comfortable and soothing for them personally. It is important never to strain the breath, and it is not necessary to ever 'suck' all the air in or to 'push' it all out. Rather, keeping the breath light and gentle during the extended inhalations or exhalations can have many physiological and emotional benefits.

It is important to practise, or to support your client to practise, any of the breathing techniques we explore in this chapter together when in a relatively balanced state (as opposed to trying them for the first time in a state of hyper- or hypo-arousal), perhaps after something relaxing like a chamomile tea or a warm bath. Making time each day, even just for a couple of minutes, to practise these techniques will help to make them readily available in the moments they are needed the most.

It is also worth mentioning that connecting to and amending the natural breathing pattern may feel very unusual and even uncomfortable for some people at first. If this is the case for you or your client, you or they might be better served by trying out the techniques and practices in other chapters before or alongside breathwork practices. (It is helpful for you as a therapist to try out these practices for yourself – they can support you personally to come into your Window of Tolerance.) Some interoceptive signals feel safer and more possible to connect with than others depending on life history, unique physiology etc. Your client might, therefore, find it helpful to connect with other interoceptive signals aside from the breath first, such as placing their hands on their heart and connecting to their heartbeat, or squeezing and releasing down their arms and legs with the hands to connect to tactile sensations. If your client feels dizzy at any point during any of the breathing practices, remind them to simply come back to long, deep breathing and take a short lie-down if possible, or to lean back in their chair.

Abdominal Breathing (also often referred to as 'diaphragmatic breathing')

It has been estimated that up to 80 per cent of people living in the Western world may be 'chest (thoracic) breathers'; they breathe predominantly using the top part of their lungs. For people experiencing anxiety, which is part and parcel of the experience of BDD, this percentage is likely to be even higher.

Importantly, the lower 10 per cent of the lungs transport more than 40 ml of oxygen per minute while the upper 10 per cent of the lungs transport less than 6 ml of oxygen per minute. That is a significant difference! The lower parts of the lungs, therefore, are around six to seven times more effective in oxygen transportation than the top of the lungs. During chest (thoracic) breathing, the lower layers of the lungs, which are more compliant ('stretchy') and more valuable in oxygen transportation, get less (if any) fresh oxygen supply. This leads to reduced cell oxygenation thus stimulating the sympathetic (fight, flight, freeze, fawn) branch of the autonomic nervous system, giving the brain the message that the person is unsafe. People who breathe thoracically are also more likely to hyperventilate, a key aspect of panic attacks.

The antidote to thoracic breathing is abdominal (diaphragmatic) breathing. A helpful beginning exercise is to invite your client to lie on their back and place one hand, fingers spread, on the abdomen and the other hand, fingers spread, on the chest reaching up to the collarbone. (They can also practise this sitting or standing if preferred; it might just be a little more difficult to sense/feel/see the movement of the abdomen.) Invite your client to breathe naturally and pay attention to the movement of their hands. Invite them to notice any movement that occurs in the abdominal and chest area during the inhalation and during the exhalation; for example, to notice whether during the inhalation the abdomen rises or falls, and whether the chest rises or falls. Is there more movement in the abdominal area (suggestive of abdominal breathing) or in the chest area (suggestive of thoracic breathing)?

Having taken note of your client's pattern of breathing, and invited them to take note also, guide your client in actively expanding their abdomen each time they take an inhalation. As they inhale, they can inflate their abdomen like a balloon. As they exhale, they can gently and lightly draw their navel in towards their spine. As a therapist, it is recommended to try diaphragmatic breathing out for yourself at least a few times, to appreciate how it feels in your own body, before supporting a client to explore the practice. You may also find this breathing helps you personally to come into your Window of Tolerance before your sessions with clients, as mentioned earlier, which will be of benefit not only to your own sense of balance but also to your client's experience of the therapeutic space.

Once your client has got the hang of expanding the abdomen on the inhalation and drawing it back towards the spine on the exhalation, they can begin to invite the breath to become a little deeper. As they inhale, they expand the abdomen and then expand the chest, sending the breath all the way up to the collarbone. Then as they exhale, they allow the collarbone to drop back, then the chest to drop back before lightly pulling in the navel towards the spine. Invite your client to notice the slight pause at the end of the exhalation before the next inhalation begins. They may notice the pause at the top of the inhalation before exhaling also.

Your client might like to try putting something onto their abdomen while lying down and practising abdominal breathing. This could be a soft toy, a stone or even a book. Invite your client to watch the stone rise each time they inhale and drop down each time they exhale. Ask them to see if they can raise the stone up nice and high as they inhale and draw it towards their spine as they come to the end of each exhalation.

Example Breathing Practices to Stimulate the Parasympathetic Branch of the Autonomic Nervous System (during times of anxiety/hyper-arousal)

In addition to lengthening the exhalation, there are other breathing practices one can engage in to stimulate the parasympathetic (energy conserving) branch of the autonomic nervous system, thus bringing one 'down' from states of anxiety and hyper-arousal. Here are a couple you might like to try with your clients.

Left-Nostril Breathing

The left nostril is linked to the right hemisphere of the brain and to the parasympathetic branch of the autonomic nervous system. Breathing through the left nostril can therefore stimulate the rest-and-digest response. Marrying this with extended exhalations (through the left nostril) can enhance this practice even further. If your client's nostrils are clear (i.e. not blocked), invite them to lightly block off the right nostril with the index finger of their right hand and breathe deeply, gently, smoothly through the left nostril, making the exhalation longer than the inhalation. Invite them to stay with the practice for at least 10–12 rounds of inhalations and exhalations to feel benefits that may last long after the practice is over.

Sitali Breath

Sitting with a lengthened spine, curl the tongue and project it around three quarters of the way out of the mouth (if one cannot curl one's tongue, simply project the tongue out of the mouth leaving a small gap between the top of the tongue and the upper lip). Inhale over the tongue as though sipping the air through a straw. Notice the pause at the top of the inhalation. Bring the tongue back into the mouth and close the lips for the exhalation, which happens through the nostrils. Notice the pause at the end of the exhalation before projecting the tongue again from the mouth to repeat the cycle.

Example Breathing Practices to Stimulate the Sympathetic Branch of the Autonomic Nervous System (during times of low mood/disaffection)

In addition to lengthening the inhalation, there are other breathing practices which can be engaged in to stimulate the sympathetic (energy mobilising) branch of the autonomic nervous system, thus bringing one 'up' from states of depression and numbness. Here are a couple you might like to try with your clients.

Right-Nostril Breathing

As in the left-nostril breathing described earlier in this chapter, although now through the right nostril which is connected to the sympathetic nervous system. Remember, this practice can be complemented and enhanced by making the inhalations longer than the exhalations to further stimulate sympathetic activity.

Breath of Fire

Breath of Fire is just as it sounds: an incredibly invigorating and stimulating breath. It is therefore definitely *not* a breathing exercise for your clients to practise in states of anxiety, but excellent at supporting an emergence from low-energy and/or depressive states.

Breath of Fire is practised through the nose. The lips remain closed, or 9/10ths closed, throughout. One makes a short, sharp exhalation through the nose as though snuffing out a candle; the inhalation then comes in without conscious effort. Each time one exhales sharply through the nose, the navel is pulled in towards the spine. Then, as the inhalation comes in of its own volition the navel moves outwards.

Breath of Fire is a rapid and rhythmic breath which is equal on the inhale and exhale with no pause between them (at around the rate of 2–3 breath cycles per second). If your client begins to feel dizzy at any point, invite them to return to long, deep breathing and take a lie down if they are able. If your client struggles with low blood pressure, is pregnant or is on the first couple of days of their menstrual cycle, the Breath of Fire may feel a little strong for them. In this case, they can stimulate their sympathetic nervous system using other breathing practices as previously described, e.g. breathing through the right nostril, extending the inhalation.

Coherent Breathing

Coherent breathing is an effective breathing practice with a growing body of research evidence behind it. For a person of average height, coherent breathing is composed of taking five diaphragmatic breaths per minute: inhaling for six seconds and exhaling for six seconds. The time interval can be adjusted depending on height (i.e. people over six feet may need longer intervals) and breath capacity. The practice can be further enhanced by lying down and placing the hands on the abdomen: expanding the abdomen on the inhalation and dropping it back towards the spine on the exhalation. There are recordings of bells, chimes etc. with time intervals of six seconds available on various music and sound platforms to support the process (search 'coherent breathing audio').

Breathing practices can be significantly beneficial for supporting the balance of the autonomic nervous system and both expanding and bringing one back into the Window of Tolerance. Inviting your clients to make the time for just a couple of minutes of breathing practices a day may make a palpable difference to their ability to cope with the anxiety and depression that are typically so much a part of the experience of BDD. Some people like to listen to music while they engage in their daily breathing practice: upbeat music alongside invigorating practices like right-nostril breathing and calming music alongside soothing practices like left-nostril breathing for example. Support your client to experiment and find what works best for them, perhaps journalling how the practices make them feel and any benefits they notice.

Your clients might find it helpful to bring these breathing practices in during necessary moments and times, for example when looking in the mirror to get ready to go out in the morning. Putting little reminders up around their living space, in their bag/pocket etc. can also be helpful. Even something as simple as the word 'breathe' painted onto a person's bathroom mirror using glass paints can be a helpful and inspiring reminder. Invite your client to be creative in how they remind themselves to use these breathing practices to support them in their journey with BDD and life in general. They can make a tangible difference.

Concluding Reflections

Considering the autonomic nervous system and HRV alongside the Window of Tolerance model and Polyvagal Theory can offer insights into the lived, embodied experience of BDD and possible avenues for soothing and healing. Associated considerations and practices can be incredibly empowering for clients, who then find they have simple tools at their fingertips for soothing themselves during times of anxiety, up-regulating themselves during times of depression and hopelessness, and staying within their Window of Tolerance if already there. Supporting clients to expand their Window of Tolerance is key, as it is here wherein emotions can be felt, expressed and processed, and feelings of a felt sense of safety in the body and the world can be experienced.

References

Corrigan, F. M., Fisher, J. J., & Nutt, D. J. (2011). Autonomic dysregulation and the window of tolerance model of the effects of complex emotional trauma. *Journal of Psychopharmacology, 25*(1), 17–25.

Dana, D. (2018). *The Polyvagal Theory in therapy: Engaging the rhythm of regulation* (Norton series on interpersonal neurobiology). WW Norton & Company.

Dana, D. (2020). *Polyvagal exercises for safety and connection: 50 client-centered practices* (Norton series on interpersonal neurobiology). WW Norton & Company.

Dana, D. (2021). *Anchored: How to befriend your nervous system using Polyvagal Theory*. Sounds True.

Ogden, P., Minton, K., & Pain, C. (2006). *Trauma and the body: A sensorimotor approach to psychotherapy* (Norton series on interpersonal neurobiology). WW Norton & Company.

Porges, S. W. (1995). Orienting in a defensive world: Mammalian modifications of our evolutionary heritage. A Polyvagal Theory. *Psychophysiology, 32*(4), 301–318.

Porges, S. W. (2011). The Polyvagal Theory: Neurophysiological foundations of emotions, attachment, communication, and self-regulation (Norton series on interpersonal neurobiology). WW Norton & Company.

Schnackenberg, N. (2019). *'The only way I was going to be lovable': A grounded theory of young people's experiences of body dysmorphic disorder* (Doctoral dissertation, University of Essex, and Tavistock and Portman NHS Foundation Trust).

Schore, A. N. (1998). Early shame experiences and infant brain development. In P. Gilbert & B. Andrews (eds), *Shame: Interpersonal behavior, psychopathology, and culture* (Series in affective science) (pp. 57–77). Oxford University Press.

Schore, A. N. (2002). Advances in neuropsychoanalysis, attachment theory, and trauma research: Implications for self psychology. *Psychoanalytic Inquiry, 22*(3), 433–484.

Siegel, D. J. (1999). *The developing mind: Toward a neurobiology of interpersonal experience*. Guilford Press.

Stern, D. N. (1985). *The interpersonal world of the infant: A view from psychoanalysis and developmental psychology*. Karnac Books.

Tomkins, S. (1963). *Affect imagery consciousness. Volume II: The negative affects*. Springer.

Chapter 9

Considering the Importance of Nutrition in BDD Recovery

———

TRISTAN KELLER

A central aspect of physical health is what we put into our bodies on a daily basis. What we eat and drink, as well as how we eat and drink, can greatly affect our physiology, as well as our capacity to handle feelings of stress, overwhelm and anxiety. In this chapter I will explore the relevance of food, eating and nutrition to the experience of body dysmorphic disorder (BDD), and offer some pointers about exploring dietary aspects with clients.

What your clients eat and drink affects their physiology and therefore their emotional state, capacity for self-regulation and so on. A nutritious diet composed also of an adequate amount and types of food can support people with BDD in handling the daily intrusive thoughts and compulsions that are so typical of the BDD experience.

We all know that nourishing the physical body optimally is easier said than done. Importantly, restrictive and rigid approaches to food and nutrition often fail, as they do not take into account a person's past history with food and eating, transgenerational narratives and aspects related to nutrition, the constant ups and downs of life and so on. It is vital to emphasise to clients that implementing a healthy diet shouldn't restrict their life but, rather, enhance it.

Experiences that sometimes go alongside BDD, like eating disorders, can have particular implications, which the scope of this chapter does not allow a nuanced exploration of. If you are working with a client who is significantly restricting their nutritional intake, it is important to signpost them towards their GP or similar for a comprehensive health check-up including an electrocardiogram and an assessment of possible electrolyte imbalances. If a person is not taking in enough nutrition or is purging the nutrition they are taking in (such as in the case of bulimia nervosa) there can be deleterious and even fatal consequences, regardless of the person's body weight.

A particularly important area to consider in the context of BDD is muscle dysmorphia. Muscle dysmorphia is a sub-type of BDD wherein a person experiences a distressing preoccupation with their musculature, typically believing themselves to be insufficiently muscular or 'puny'. People experiencing muscle dysmorphia may cut whole food groups out of their diet (e.g. carbohydrates), exercise excessively (including beyond the point of physical exhaustion and during times of injury) and ingest protein powders and/or anabolic steroids or similar in an attempt to increase their muscle mass. Again, if working therapeutically with a client with muscle dysmorphia it is important to have their physical health checked by a qualified medical practitioner.

An important aspect of therapy for people experiencing BDD is the development of a more self-compassionate, meaningful and flexible approach to health, including in relation to nutrition and exercise. An overarching concept for therapists to consider when working with clients with BDD is to emphasise the function of the body over the form – exploring what the body can do and how it feels as opposed to how it looks. Any approach to exploring food and exercise can helpfully begin from this premise also, i.e. exercise undertaken in order to feel better rather than to lose weight; foods chosen because they promote health and make the person feel good as opposed to being chosen because they are low in calories etc.

Some people with BDD have a difficult and pained relationship with food and eating. They may restrict their diet to change the shape of a particular body part (for example, to change the shape of their legs or their face), eat only certain foods to prevent their skin from becoming blemished or their teeth becoming yellow and so on. Part of the therapeutic process very often, therefore, is supporting clients to nurture a comfortable relationship with food and eating. The involvement of a dietician and/or nutritionist can sometimes be helpful in this process.

Shame, Emotional Regulation and Food
Overeating, undereating, drinking alcohol excessively, smoking and the use of illegal drugs in the context of BDD are often the result of an

inability to tolerate intense feelings of shame, anxiety, fear, anger and overwhelm. Sometimes, such as in the case of drinking alcohol and using illegal substances, they are used to facilitate social interactions, e.g. feeling unable to go into a social situation due to intense anxiety related to the preoccupation with aspects of the appearance unless intoxicated with alcohol.

An important aspect of therapy for BDD, therefore, is supporting clients to develop a capacity to tolerate, feel and ideally embrace their emotions and bodily sensations. They can be supported to inquire, with curiosity and compassion, into why they make the choices they make regarding food, nutrition, exercise and so on and consider how other options may better serve them. It can be helpful to explore with clients:

- What emotions are present when you abstain from eating, eat to excess etc.?

- When you abstain from eating for example, what are you striving towards or hoping for?

- What are you trying to change (internally and externally) when you purge away the food you have eaten?

- When you exercise excessively, what is your motivation?

- What do you feel drinking alcohol, taking drugs etc. facilitates for you?

Shame typically begets shame, therefore emotional repression or acting on compulsions are common mechanisms of coping for people experiencing BDD. Clients with BDD can helpfully be supported to validate their emotions, including by experiencing them with compassion towards themselves, while inquiring with genuine curiosity into what their meaning might be. Rather than fighting their thoughts and compulsions, it's essential for people experiencing BDD to acknowledge their feelings and bodily sensations, including an exploration of what these feelings and bodily sensations might be trying to tell them: their message and 'story'. Other chapters in this book explore these ideas further: for example, Rosa Hernando Hontoria's chapter on Compassion Focused Therapy (Chapter 11) and the Schnackenbergs' chapter on Voice Dialogue (Chapter 13).

It is helpful to support clients to find ways to take a moment to feel into their emotions before acting on their compulsions, such as the compulsion to exercise or restrict their diet. This will help clients to feel less like victims of their compulsions, and to be able to embrace their emotional pain, rather than trying to escape from it (with courage and understanding).

While psychological flexibility, non-judgmental awareness and self-compassion skills are essential to establishing a healthy relationship with food and oneself, I would like to turn now to more concrete matters concerning nutritional and behavioural advice. The question remains: what kind of diet could be conducive to recovery from BDD? How and what can people experiencing BDD eat and drink to feel more stable, energised and grounded?

The goal (which may, in some cases, be supported by the involvement of a certified dietician or nutritionist) is to find a nutritional approach that first and foremost supplies a person with enough energy to maintain emotional stability throughout the day, while avoiding foods and substances that destabilise the mood or negatively impact upon emotional regulation. Importantly, any nutritional approach should be designed to work for a person in the long term, enhancing wellbeing and quality of life both presently and into the future.

Glycaemic Index and Sugar

Emotional regulation is significantly supported by keeping blood sugars relatively steady throughout the day. This includes the avoidance of insulin-spiking foods as these can negatively impact upon energy levels and, therefore, one's ability to cope with the intrusive thoughts and compulsions characteristic of BDD. It is supportive for clients to eat regular meals composed of whole, unprocessed or minimally processed foods which are low on the glycaemic index and include a source of protein, e.g. rolled oats with nut milk, sweet potatoes with chickpeas, eggs on wholegrain toast, cheese and apple chunks, green vegetables with wholegrain pasta, brown rice and fish. This will reduce or even eliminate the blood-sugar highs and lows which come from skipping meals or consuming sugary or highly processed foods. It may be helpful to share with clients that high blood sugar levels can affect the ability of the hippocampus to react to stress.

It can be beneficial to support clients with BDD to keep a diary relating what they eat, and how and when they eat, to experiences related to BDD. For example, they may like to look for correlations between what they eat and how they feel; when they exercise and the BDD-related compulsions; how hungry they are and how they feel about their appearance and so on. Studies have demonstrated that people with BDD may have differential interoceptive awareness (the lived experience of the body from the inside) in some areas than people without BDD, as explored in more detail in Nicole Schnackenberg's chapter on the brain and sensory system (Chapter 5). Hunger and fullness are interoceptive signals also. Poor interoception regarding hunger and fullness levels can easily lead to skipped meals or regularly eating beyond the point of fullness. It is important for people experiencing BDD, therefore, to be supported to connect with and develop their interoceptive awareness. Approaches such as yoga and mindfulness meditation, as explored in chapters elsewhere in this book, can be helpful in this process.

The Brain in the Gut

Professor David Veale, one of the leading experts and researchers in BDD, appreciates the gut–brain connection for psychological wellbeing, including in the context of BDD (Veale & Mitchell, 2021). Of particular interest to Veale and others is the gut microbiome: the ecosystem of the bacteria, fungi and viruses living in the gut of every human being. An important aspect is the relationship this gut microbiome has with the brain, known as the 'gut–brain axis' or, more colloquially, 'the brain in the gut'. The gut and brain are linked via the vagus nerve, which is part of the autonomic nervous system. Additionally, there is a local nervous system in the gut itself which operates independently to the brain: the enteric nervous system (sometimes referred to as the 'second brain'). The enteric nervous system also receives brain signals via the vagus nerve.

How the gut microbiome in each individual person is made up depends on the unique ecosystem of microbes they were born with, which is initially influenced by the microbiota of the mother. Throughout the lifespan this microbiota is influenced, changes and develops depending on both genetic and lifestyle factors, notably the diet. Importantly, the ecosystem of the gut has been demonstrated to impact upon the brain through the levels of chemicals which influence it. This affects mood and general wellbeing. The relationship is a two-way street: psychological distress can influence the gut microbiome also.

Clients can get an idea of the composition of their microbiota by sending a sample of their faeces off for analysis to one of many companies across the UK and worldwide who offer this service. When recommend-ing such a company to your client, ensure they are reputable, seeking professional recommendation where possible. Your client should then receive guidance, specific to the composition of their unique microbiome, about which foods and nutritional approach may be the most and least supportive. General dietary guidelines in terms of supporting a diverse and healthy gut microbiome include, but are certainly not limited to:

- Introduction of probiotics.

- Ingestion of probiotic foods, for example fermented foods (e.g. sauerkraut and kefir).

- Ingestion of prebiotic foods, for example many unprocessed plant-based foods (e.g. lentils, beans and broccoli).

- Aiming for 50 different vegetables, legumes, grains, nuts, fruits and herbs each week (Professor David Veale, alongside others, rec-ommends starting with a target of 30 and building up gradually).

- Inclusion of polyphenols (responsible for the bright colours of fruits and vegetables, i.e. 'eating the rainbow').

- Swapping white/brown bread for sourdough bread to increase intake of prebiotic fibre and polyphenols.

Caffeine and Alcohol

As part of our discussion, it is important to consider two other key factors which can physiologically impact upon one's ability to process and regulate emotions, including impacting on the gut microbiome, namely alcohol and caffeine. While both alcohol and caffeine seem to have become dietary staples in the Western world for some, excessive consumption can considerably hinder the BDD recovery process.

In the case of caffeine, excessive consumption can overstimulate the regions of the brain responsible for threat perception. This can heighten one's susceptibility to experiencing anxiety and BDD-associated safety behaviours. Your client may have noticed, for example, that when they drink too much coffee or another caffeinated beverage, they become more easily startled, jittery, agitated or feel more anxious. Concerning the quantity, most studies indicate that consuming more than 400 mg of caffeine per day is associated with significant increases in anxiety, while the results for quantities between 100 mg and 400 mg per day are mixed. Herbal teas or chicory root 'coffee' are alternatives which are typically caffeine free, e.g. chamomile tea, fennel tea, ginger tea.

Another downside of caffeine is its impact on sleep, both the ease of falling asleep and sleep quality. Studies are increasingly demonstrating how the quality of one's sleep is vital for several processes linked to health, longevity, optimal psychological functioning and wellbeing. Therefore, it is helpful to support clients to consider cutting back on caffeine consumption in general, but especially in the afternoon when caffeine is most likely to have a negative impact on sleep and to disrupt sleeping patterns.

The half-life of caffeine ranges between five and seven hours: five to seven hours after drinking coffee, there is still 50 per cent of the initial caffeine dose circulating through the brain tissue. Sharing this information with clients with BDD can be very helpful when compiling a plan together for gradually cutting down caffeine consumption. It is important to be mindful that caffeine is present in other products also, e.g. chocolate and cola.

It can be helpful to share with clients how excessive caffeine consumption can create a vicious cycle. By impairing one's ability to fall asleep, as well as affecting the quality of sleep, a person can be left feeling tired and 'on edge' the next day. As a consequence, the person may feel they just 'need' some coffee to get them through the morning or day. It can also be helpful to share with clients how the nervous system habituates to input from stimulants such as caffeine, e.g. gradually, more and more caffeine is required for the same alerting effects over time. Therefore, what might start off as one coffee mid-morning as a 'pick-me-up' may rapidly become two or three coffees, or coffees consumed throughout the day.

In the case of alcohol, the picture is similar to that of caffeine, although caffeine is a stimulant while alcohol is, essentially, a depressant. It is the quantity, timing and frequency of your client's consumption of alcohol in the short and long term which is important to address. Again, alcohol can have a deleterious impact upon the quality of one's sleep, which can destabilise mood the following day.

Alcohol has especially detrimental effects on REM sleep, which is essential for the overnight processing of experienced emotions and memories, as well as to the ability to read and comprehend emotional cues from others. For example, in a study wherein they explored how sleep impacts upon the ability to accurately assess the emotional quality of facial expressions, participants who were deprived of REM-sleep were more easily threatened by even gentle or friendly looking faces (Van Der Helm, Gujar & Walker, 2010). As we know, the threat-detection system in BDD tends to typically be in hyper-alert, as people with BDD often scan the faces of others assuming they will react in the same disgust to their physical appearance as they do themselves.

It is common knowledge that alcohol can help people to 'loosen' up, feel more jovial and relaxed, and increase feelings of social confidence. For these benefits, alcohol is understandably popular, and especially in the West, it is typically an integrated aspect of many social occasions and festivities. For people experiencing BDD, however, alcohol can become problematic when it is used to cope with overwhelming emotions, such as shame or social anxiety. Habitual, excessive alcohol use deprives one of the opportunity to experience, feel and tolerate one's emotions, which is an essential part of healing from any emotional struggle – and BDD is no exception. Therefore, it can be helpful to consider with clients whether they are using alcohol for enjoyment or to cope with uncomfortable or overwhelming emotions including experiences of social anxiety, and whether the use of alcohol is serving them in the short and/or long term.

Personally, I don't believe in rigid diets and restrictions, therefore I'm not suggesting advocating to clients with BDD that they cut out caffeine and alcohol completely, though there may be some cases where this is helpful, even vital. In general, healthy living is about striking a balance and finding out what works best for a person in the long term. However, if your client feels stuck with their BDD compulsions and intrusive thoughts and feelings, and they are regularly experiencing high levels of agitation, anxiety and/or depression throughout the day, it may be helpful to take a close look at the consumption of alcohol and caffeine and consider if some significant changes may be supportive and necessary.

Allergies, Intolerances and Deficiencies

It is also important to consider allergies and deficiencies in the context of BDD. Alongside possible gastrointestinal symptoms, deficiencies and/or allergies can also reinforce neurologic and psychiatric symptoms if they remain undiagnosed and untreated. Allergies exist on a spectrum, ranging from mild sensitivities to extreme allergic reactions.

Allergies can affect one's physical and mental resiliency in the context of BDD. It is worth considering with clients whether allergies and/or intolerances may be impacting upon their wellbeing, and also on their sense of self. Even a mild sensitivity can leave a person feeling dizzy and lethargic throughout the day. Ruling out any allergies is important when working with BDD, as indeed it is with any mental health struggle. Referral for allergy/sensitivity/intolerance testing may be appropriate and supportive in some cases.

Nutritional deficiencies can also have deleterious impacts on a person's physical health and emotional wellbeing. A folate (vitamin B9) deficiency, for example, is associated with higher rates of depression. Again, referral to a GP or similar may be appropriate, especially if a client is presenting as exhausted despite adequate sleep, with dark circles under the eyes, notably pale and with issues such as especially dry or chapped skin, dry and brittle hair, dizziness etc.

The Mediterranean Diet

While many dietary approaches advocate restricting or forbidding certain food groups, it is my personal belief that this approach can ultimately prove to be futile in the long run. Rather than following a specific or restrictive diet, it is perhaps more sensible and beneficial to follow a diet which supports one's mental health and physical longevity, while at the same time being (at least relatively) easy to implement.

With regards to mental health, a dietary approach where supportive evidence has been found in reducing depressive symptoms is the Mediterranean diet (for example, Godos et al., 2018). A major reason why the Mediterranean diet can be conducive to one's mental health and wellbeing is due to its relatively low amount of the foods that could potentially impede emotional stability (sugars, high glycaemic foods etc.) and its inclusion of many foods which are beneficial for emotional stability (unprocessed vegetables, low glycaemic foods, fish etc.).

While the Mediterranean diet is low in many of the foods which have become staples in the typical Western diet, e.g. simple sugars, high glycaemic foods, processed foods and saturated fats, no food groups are 'forbidden' per se. This gives the Mediterranean diet a certain flexibility, as well as applicability in different social and cultural contexts.

Concerning its composition, the Mediterranean diet consists primarily of unprocessed vegetables, fresh fruits, nuts and seeds, whole grains, fish and healthy oils, particularly olive oil. It contains low to moderate amounts of red meat, egg and dairy products, which are consumed occasionally. Sugary treats and confectionaries are not 'forbidden', but they are viewed as an exception or infrequent addition, rather than consumed daily.

A diet composed of unprocessed vegetables, legumes and whole grains may help people experiencing BDD to be less likely to fall prey to intrusive thoughts and BDD compulsions. At the same time, it will likely supply them with ample energy to optimally use the tools and insights acquired in therapy, further supporting self-regulation skills and improving a felt sense of agency.

Importantly, diets high in monounsaturated fatty acids (as found in olive oil and almonds), as well as polyunsaturated fatty acids (as found in fish and walnuts), have been found to reduce the risk of depression. Especially Omega 3 fatty acids, which are mostly found in seafood, have strong anti-inflammatory properties and seem to have a positive effect on many mental health conditions, ranging from ADHD (attention deficit hyperactivity disorder) to PTSD (post-traumatic stress disorder).

Containing plenty of healthy oils, nuts, seeds and fish, the Mediter-ranean diet provides a sufficient supply of healthy fats throughout the day to support optimal neurological functioning. As someone with lived experience of BDD, I can personally and very highly attest to the physical and psychological benefits of eating this way.

Concluding Reflections

While these small, daily dietary choices may seem trivial at first, I earnestly believe proper nutrition matters in the long term. Improper nutrition can leave anyone, including people experiencing BDD, feeling more agitated, stressed and anxious, therefore posing an impediment to the recovery process. Optimal, or at least improved, nutrition can be significantly supportive to emotional stability, enhanced mood and better sleep.

It is vital for therapists working with BDD to hold in mind that any self-negating behaviours related to food and eating are highly likely to stem from unprocessed traumatic experiences and may be the client's current means to self-regulate. Therefore, any nutritional changes will be extremely difficult to implement if the underlying emotional landscape is left unaddressed, and other means of emotional regulation and soothing are not explored.

With regards to the light-touch nutritional advice offered in this chapter, I think it is sensible to introduce just one, or maximum two, dietary measurements and try them out for two to three weeks, to assess for any changes such as improved mood or enhanced emotional well-being. Introducing changes one-by-one will make it easier to discern any causal relationship between your client's diet and their psychological wellbeing. Making just one or two changes will also likely feel more possible and manageable for your client, rather than inviting lots of changes at one and the same time.

Concerning the nutritional changes themselves, striving for effectiveness is key. I feel there is perhaps little merit in turning the diet of your client upside down if the results with regards to emotional stability and wellbeing are meagre. The goal is not merely to introduce 'a healthier diet' to your client, but rather to explore possible dietary changes that may support your client in their recovery process. This approach necessarily involves gently and regularly enquiring, with openness and curiosity, about their dietary habits, including exploring any which may be impeding their recovery journey. It is reasonable, I feel, to ask from time to time, particularly if your client experiences an extreme episode of shame or a BDD 'flare-up', what they have been eating or drinking that day or week. You may discover that your client has not eaten enough, didn't sleep well or has been using stimulants or sedatives the day/week before the 'flare-up'. While correlation certainly doesn't prove causation, and many other aspects may also be at play, considering the impact of possible dietary elements alongside other factors can be highly beneficial.

Experience is the best teacher. If your client experiences the mood-stabilising, resilience-enhancing benefits of optimal (or at least improved) nutrition, the motivational benefits that may lead to lasting change will, I believe, likely come.

References

Godos, J., Castellano, S., Ray, S., Grosso, G., & Galvano, F. (2018). Dietary polyphenol intake and depression: Results from the Mediterranean healthy eating, lifestyle and aging (meal) study. *Molecules, 23*(5), 999.

Van Der Helm, E., Gujar, N., & Walker, M. P. (2010). Sleep deprivation impairs the accurate recognition of human emotions. *Sleep, 33*(3), 335–342.

Veale, D., & Mitchell, V. (2021) How eating nutrient-dense foods might improve your brain health. Accessed 13/11/2022 at www.veale.co.uk/news/eating-nutrient-dense-foods-might-improve-brain-health

Chapter 10

Considering Acceptance and Commitment Therapy in the Context of BDD

SARAH SIVERS

This chapter explores some central ideas connected to Acceptance and Commitment Therapy (ACT). It offers sample activities to bring key ACT ideas to life, inviting a different way of thinking about and working with BDD.

This offering is not intended as a comprehensive overview of ACT as a therapeutic model. ACT has many layers – practical and theoretical – which go beyond the scope of this chapter. The aim here is to offer an overview of key ACT concepts which can be used with creativity, individuality and curiosity. It is hoped this may prompt the start of a journey to an ACT-informed and meaningful way of interacting with the experience of BDD.

The activities and ideas offered here have been shared in a BDD support group and adapted and added to following feedback from experts-by-lived-experience of BDD. ACT resonates and works for me and others I have shared it with. It will not work for everyone and that's okay. The most important thing is to give it a go with an open heart and curious mind.

A Brief Overview of What ACT Is and Isn't

ACT was first developed by clinical psychologist Steven Hayes and colleagues (Hayes, Strosahl & Wilson, 1999) as part of what has been named a third wave in behavioural and cognitive therapies. ACT has been adapted and extended since to offer support to children, adolescents and adults by way of providing an alternative way of managing the ups and downs of life.

Some initial research has been conducted to explore how ACT can be used to support those experiencing BDD, for example, a pilot project exploring a group intervention (Linde et al., 2015), some case studies (Dehbaneh, 2019) and a client interview following ACT (Pickard, Lumby & Deane, 2021). A consistent conclusion from these studies was that BDD-related worries and feelings of shame were reduced and interpersonal relationships and quality of life increased following a series of sessions of ACT. Key components of positive change were suggested to be connected with the values-based approach and the modelling of acceptance which is inherent to ACT. A reference list is provided at the end of this chapter for those interested in reading about the various applications and psychological underpinnings of ACT further.

ACT is an active way to approach life. This is one of the reasons why those who have developed ACT emphasise that it should be pronounced as the word 'act', rather than A-C-T: to illuminate the way we can act in a mindful way, with meaning (Harris, 2019). One of the most powerful psychological processes within ACT, and one which may potentially resonate with those experiencing BDD, is that of acceptance. ACT acknowledges and seeks to support individuals to accept that difficult thoughts and emotions are part of life. The work, therefore, focuses on how a person notices and responds to, rather than trying to eliminate or change, thought patterns and ideas.

ACT provides techniques and thinking tools to support an individual in acknowledging they have some agency in when and how BDD shows up. ACT is not a magic wand: it takes work and thought, which leads us onto the commitment element. Part of the work (the commitment made) is how to move towards a values-guided life, particularly as there is the hope that this might also include, one day, looking at the value or values BDD itself may hold. This approach is all undertaken with curiosity and creativity.

Core Tenets of ACT

Some of the central tenets of ACT are the ideas of psychological flexibility and being 'open, aware and active'. See the following figure for a visual representation of psychological flexibility, commonly known as the Hexaflex model (Wilson & DuFrene, 2008). This model encompasses six core processes that guide a person to engage with the world in a more flexible way. These ideas interlink with each other, and each element can be brought to the forefront depending on what would be useful to explore or engage with. The beauty of ACT is that this is thought about in practical and creative ways.

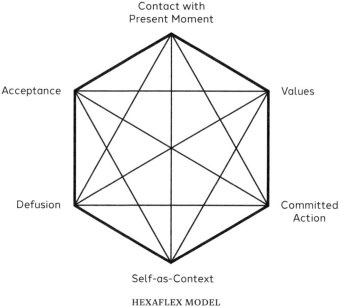

HEXAFLEX MODEL
Adapted from Wilson & DuFrene (2008)[1]

Open, Aware and Active

The six psychological flexibility processes within the Hexaflex model are interconnected with one's ability to be open, aware and active in how one engages with life experiences. These concepts of openness, awareness and activeness are often referred to as the three pillars of wellbeing (Gillard & Brown, 2016):

- *Open*: Welcoming life and what it brings in a heartfelt way.

- *Aware*: Noticing experiences, thoughts, feelings, memories and embodied sense of being.

1   Original copyright © Steven C. Hayes. Used with permission.

- *Active*: Doing things that matter and being guided by and living in tune with one's values.

Defusion
To understand the concept of defusion, it is helpful to first consider the psychological theory ACT is based on, that of Relational Frame Theory (RTF) (Hayes, Barnes-Holmes and Roche, 2013).

Relational Frame Theory
RTF is a psychological theory of human language and cognition which attempts to explain how language-able humans generate meaning and understanding in the world (Hayes et al., 2013). From an RFT perspective, the meaning of a particular thought or verbal utterance is determined by the context in which it arises. In the early learning of language this context is direct learning from a language-adept other, i.e. a caregiver who names objects and enables connection between an arbitrary word (collection of sounds) and the object. This direct connection between object and word can also be taught and learned by other animals (e.g. a dog reacting to the word 'walk'). However, as language-able children develop, they derive more complex relationships from the directly learned relations, that is, to make connections which are not directly taught (known as derived relational responding (DRR)).

To illustrate the difference between directly learned relations and DRR: if a child (or indeed adult) is taught that a is taller than b, b is taller than c, c is taller than d and d is taller than e, that individual has been taught four direct relations (in this case, size-comparison relations). They will also likely begin to make other connections from this information, for example deriving that a is taller than c. This is the wonder of DRR in action. This DRR process can be applied to more complex relational frames. Just imagine how much of our language is the result of DRR, rather than directly learned experiences!

A critical feature and assumption of RFT is that learning (including learning language relations) works by addition not subtraction. There are also limitless relational frames one can create (and add to), which are given even more meaning by one's embodied and emotional experience connected with these frames. This adds even more resonance to why, when a person learns or derives a particular relation, they can't just take it out and start again. The way in which relations become embedded (and automatic) can be experienced by engaging in the quiz below, an exercise you might like to try with your clients experiencing BDD by way of psychoeducation on RFT in action.

Relational Frame Quiz
Try to stop yourself from automatically filling in the blanks

1. Once upon a . . . .

2. One, two, ..., four, five

3. Ready, steady . . . .

4. I am . . . .

5. Arctic . . . .

Context, of course, matters with one's responses to the quiz. Regardless, this short exercise demonstrates how quickly and automatically links can come up within thought. It perhaps also supports reflection on how relational frames can't just be 'taken out' (directly learned or derived) in order to 'start again'. This has particularly important implications for therapeutic work, including in the context of BDD.

Part of the ACT journey is to become more mindful of these relational frames; to take the time to step back and question the automatic links a person has made; and to be more flexible with one's thinking. In fact, all of the six therapeutic processes articulated in the ACT Hexaflex have been developed based on RFT. Let's take a look at these in more depth, starting on the left of the Hexaflex with defusion and working round.

Defusing Thoughts

Defusion invites a person to stand back and observe their thoughts in order to mindfully explore if they are helpful or not. Defusion is the counterbalance to fused thoughts, which are those thoughts which are fixed and may focus on absolutes: *I am ugly… I only need to fix my nose in order to feel good about myself… I always disgust people with my appearance… I never appear attractive to others…*etc. Fused thoughts are relational frames which have become embedded and automatic. These fused thoughts are also very often self-critical in nature.

The function of defusion in ACT is to gently question fused thoughts, rather than being caught up with them, and to explore if these thoughts are helpful in a given moment and if they are working in one's favour. An exercise to encourage this gentle questioning is outlined below.

Defusion Exercise

Invite your client to try out this exercise during the experience of a rumination on a negative or uncomfortable thought or experience:

Catch the thought and think or say aloud, 'I am having a fused thought.'

Take a deep breath and think or say, 'I am thinking I am...' and then extend this to 'I am noticing a thought that...'

Take another deep breath and gently ask, 'Is this thought working for me (in a life-affirming and supportive way)?'

Consider if this thought is in sync with identified values: 'Is this thought that I have noticed helping me to fulfil my values?'

Acceptance

It is important to note that at no point in the defusion exercise is the emphasis on proving the thought wrong, trying to change it or removing it. The thought is merely there; it can be considered and looked at, believed or not believed, followed and acted upon or not. This type of flexible thinking reflects the acceptance element of the ACT Hexaflex. However, in ACT, acceptance does not suggest that the thoughts are simply to be tolerated or that a person should passively accept their situation as it is. Acceptance in ACT is active with curiosity and openness to what is happening, including to the painful and difficult experiences and aspects of life over which one has little or no control (the past, the actions of others, one's height, skin tone etc.). Acceptance in ACT is about making room for all of life's experiences, rather than striving to fight or resist them (Harris, 2019).

Self-as-Context

In ACT, the self-as-context process is the awareness of what one is thinking, feeling or experiencing at any given time. It is not the 'self-story' but an 'observing self' or the part that notices (Harris, 2019, p. 7).

Contact with the Present Moment

The processes we have considered so far – defusion, acceptance, self-as-context and now contact with the present moment – are all viewed as mindfulness-focused processes within ACT. Contact with the present moment literally means being in the moment, and actively paying attention to what is happening and therefore engaging in an active, open and aware way to one's present experiences. This links with the idea of attentional refocusing which Rob Willson explores in Chapter 14.

Committed Action

The final two processes of the ACT Hexaflex focus on more active elements of engaging with the world. Committed action refers to doing what it takes to engage in a more rich and meaningful life. This might be supporting your client to set targets and plan actions in relation to their experience of BDD, doing so in a mindful and committed way. Committed action is also guided by one's values.

Values

The values element allows an exploration of the things that matter most to a person and how these values can guide one's actions.

Values are actions and intentions which hold meaning and importance for us. People have different values and tend to associate different values with different situations. However, there are usually a few guiding values or principles individuals hold very dear which are vitally important to them. These values can guide and comfort, support the making of decisions and leverage a person in moving towards or away from situations in their lives.

Exploring Values

Please see Appendix A for a longer list of values. On the next page is an example of a shorter list you might like to use as a starter for this exercise with your client. It is important to let your client know that they should feel at liberty to add their own values as the lists are not exhaustive: each person is very likely to have ideas which are unique to them! This is also an activity you can do in relation to your own personal values as a therapist.

Honesty	Acceptance	Self-Care
To be honest, truthful and sincere with myself and others	To be open to and allowing of things I don't want or dislike in myself, others and the world around me	To care for and be kind to myself; to allow myself time to rest and recharge
Playfulness	**Trust**	**Creativity**
To be playful, creative and light hearted in my approach to life; to see the joy in playful moments	To be trustworthy, loyal, faithful, sincere and reliable; also, to be trusting of others	To be creative and innovative at work and play; to enjoy and promote the creativity of others
Nurture	**Curiosity**	**Courage**
To care for and hold in mind those around me and myself; to protect and keep others and myself safe	To be curious, open-minded and interested; eager to explore, discover and learn new things	To be courageous or brave; to persist in the face of fear, uncertainty and threatening circumstances

Invite your client to take some time to actively think about each value in the list in front of them; they might take a few hours or days to do this, or it may be something they want to do quickly and instinctively to start with during a therapeutic session or at home. Ask your client to think about how they might order the values. One suggestion is to create a pile of: those which are important or resonate; those which do so to a lesser degree; and some 'Maybes' or 'Sometimes'. Invite your client to sort the values in a way which best works for them.

Invite your client to start with the pile of values which speak to and/ or are important or noteworthy for them. They may only have a couple in their pile or they may have many. Invite them to spend some time picking out the three key values which mean the most to them at this moment in their lives. Your client can keep the other piles they have made; they will look at them again later.

Now your client has three key values which are important to them. If the client has not already chosen it, invite them to find the self-care value card and add to the three they have picked. For many people struggling with BDD this isn't one they tend to choose. You might like to tell them that this is the value you offer to them to invite nurture into their life, alongside the values they may have chosen in relation to caring for, being kind to and thinking of others. Your client may have chosen the nurturing card; it can be helpful to wonder with them whether they registered that it also asks them to nurture themselves.

The next step is to move forwards with those three key values and explore how else ACT can help soothe and support one's journey.

Exploring Chosen Values

ACT invites us to be creative and indeed playful about the way we view and interact with the world. Therefore, as well as thinking about one's key values in relation to the practical aspects of what they mean to and/ or bring to one's life, these values can also be brought to life in a playful way, even inviting some humour and imagination into the process of owning one's values.

People don't have to stay with the same values in all situations and through different times in their lives. Different values are needed and drawn upon for different situations. Invite your client to return to the piles of values they sorted in the first exercise and to look at the values which didn't make the 'Important' pile (or the name they gave to the values that resonated least for them). Next, invite them to look at some of these and spend a bit of time thinking about why they did not stand out for them. Your client may like to consider the following questions:

- What is it about this value that didn't resonate with me?

- Is this a value I think I can't achieve or do?

- Is it a value I would like to have?

- Is it a value I associate with someone else? How?

- Could I try on this value and see what it would be like to use it? Where would it show up?

- What would I notice myself doing differently if this value were to be part of my life?

- How might my experience of my appearance/BDD be different if this value were part of my day-to-day living?

It can be illuminating to examine BDD through a values lens. You can support your client to discover what values they can find embedded within the BDD experience which could be directed outwards and used less painfully, in a more life-giving way. It may be, for example, that they are very *creative* or *innovative* with make-up and clothing: that *eye for detail* could be beneficial when looking out on the world and seeing what could be changed, when engaging in creative and artistic pursuits and so on. This is a theme we will touch on too in the 'Passengers on the Bus' activity later in this chapter. Ideas related to defusion could also be helpful here, e.g. *I am noticing an aspect of perfectionism in BDD – there is value to perfectionism; how else could this perfectionism be used to help me move towards [whatever it is]?*

Trying on Different Values

This activity focuses on inviting your client to try taking on a different value; to try out a different way of being, maybe a value that is not embedded in or directed by BDD. This activity brings into play all six processes of the ACT Hexaflex and encourages an open, active and aware exploration of alternative values. While this thinking about values does not directly focus on changing specific aspects of the BDD, values-driven actions and values exploration can offer an alternative way of being and thinking. This may then be transferred to how one views and manages BDD; or a more values-driven approach to life may shift BDD to the back of the bus, a metaphor we will explore later in more depth. For example, your client might like to consider what it would be like to explore and bring into their life the value of playfulness. How and where could this value be brought into their day-to-day experience? What might it look like? Feel like? How might the value of playfulness serve to relax the anxious thoughts about their appearance? And so on.

Keeping Values Front and Centre

A way to keep one's values at the forefront of how one lives one's life is to have gentle reminders around. A simple and effective way to do this is by using the thing many of us have close to us a lot of the time – our phone.

Most of us have at least a few images on our phone. We are not talking about photographs of the self here, which can be triggering and difficult for clients with BDD to look at, but rather images of plants, landscapes, animals etc. With this activity, you can invite your client to have one of their core values in mind and to then open up their images app on their phone (or something like Google Images if they prefer), and scroll through. Invite them to stop when they get to an image which resonates with the value they are holding in mind. It might be an obvious association or something more abstract.

If your client can't find an image that works, they might start by looking around for a way to represent this value. They can be as literal or as abstract as they wish to be. They may collect up various images for different values. They may even wish to draw, collage or sculpt their values.

Next, invite your client to take this image and put it somewhere they can see it regularly, for example to set it as their background or lockscreen or to print it out and have it on their wall, in their bag/wallet.

Invite your client to spend some time every day with these visual representations of their values in a mindful way. It may also be helpful to them to have some space for reflection at the beginning of the day, the end of the day or both. Your client may like to use this time to think about how they will use or have used these values that day, what they have brought to them and others, and how they may keep bringing this value into their life.

BDD through a Values Lens

The experience of BDD can be all-encompassing: it can leave a person feeling as though it is difficult or even impossible to think about anything else. Supporting your client to find a way of having a short amount of time – even 30 seconds or less – to bring their mind and heart to their underlying values may help them to shift away from the BDD-related thoughts and give their inner cheerleader a chance to flourish their pom-pom.

Some people find it helpful to conceptualist BDD as a frightened part or aspect of the self which also has protective elements, and is yearning to be both understood and nurtured. It might be helpful to support your client to consider how they conceptualise BDD: As a persecutory bully? As a frightened child? As an energetic protector? Something else? The Compassion Focused Therapy chapter (Chapter 11) and the Voice Dialogue chapter (Chapter 13) within this book may be helpful in supporting you and your client to think more about this.

Introducing Psychological Flexibility through the 'Passengers on the Bus' Metaphor

Metaphor is often used as a tool to explore thoughts and experiences in a creative way within the ACT framework. A classic metaphor in ACT is that of the 'Passengers on the Bus'. This activity invites a person to take notice of their multi-faceted lives through imagining themselves as the driver of a bus, with a range of passengers who may make the journey easier or more difficult. This metaphor-based activity invites a person to be more open, aware and active in thinking about what is happening for them in the present moment. It encourages a noticing of the self-in-context and is an invitation to engage in defusion, alongside an exploration of values, which then can lead to committed action. There is also the invitation to accept all the passengers who join the bus and to be open to the purpose they may play in the journey forward.

The bus can be seen as the container for all the person's thoughts, feelings and values; these are the passengers. If your client thinks back to the last time they were on an actual bus, I wonder if they looked around at the passengers: Were they all the same? Did some stand out?

In your client's bus they have all the passengers they have collected over time – some might have been with them for a very long time and be very familiar. There may be new passengers who have recently stepped on. There will be passengers yet to be collected or who have maybe been driven past because the bus felt too full.

As the driver, your client decides the journey and destination. Support them to consider that they may have become stuck on tried-and-tested routes, even if they are not interesting or lifegiving and don't take them anywhere – this could be seen as an everlasting ring-road going round and round. There may be very vocal passengers on their bus encouraging them to keep to this route; they may do so in a reassuring or a bullying way. These passengers may have names like 'worry', the 'unfavourable comparer', 'pessimism', 'perfectionist', 'BDD', 'kindness', 'clarity' and 'connection'. These passengers can be nervous, scared, empowering or protective at different times and in different situations.

One day your client might pick up a new passenger – let's call them 'the rebel' – and they want to shake things up a bit. They suggest your client takes a turn off the tried-and-tested route to explore somewhere new! This is when the old and familiar passengers might start to make a noise and to tell your client all the reasons why they should not make the change. There can be lots of passengers against one...what to do?!

There are many answers to this question:

- Your client might decide to stay with the tried-and-tested routes, to let 'the rebel' off at the next stop and make sure they don't take on any passengers like that again.

- Your client may try to battle it out with the grumpy, scared and negative passengers, but this might take all of their energy, leaving them feeling like the destination is not worth it in the end.

- Your client may listen to 'the rebel' but not heed some of the more cautious passengers. This might result in their going too far off their route or getting lost (too far from their values).

- Or... (and this is where the ACT Hexaflex processes come in) your client may accept that this noise – the babble of the various passengers – is just there. They may choose not to fight it, and equally not to let it overwhelm them. You might support your client to listen to their various passengers and think about how they can work with these thoughts – some of the 'complaining passengers' may actually be useful – reminding your client of their core values and stopping them from going too far off track. For example, a passenger might offer a protective presence, stopping your client from being too rebellious and getting into lots of trouble!

BDD will be a passenger on this bus and one that may seem to command and direct at all times (a backseat driver). Your client may have a particular name or names for their experience of BDD, which might show up in different ways as different passengers for them at different times. It may be helpful to support your client to notice that BDD does not need to take up all of the space on the bus, or indeed be in the driver's seat all, or perhaps even in any of the seats at different times. It can be helpful to support your client to sit with the BDD passenger(s) for a while and wonder what elements of value they offer or guide them towards; what underlying protective presence is offered? This is where the concept of defusion can support and guide your client's thinking and curiosity about BDD. What questions might they ask BDD and indeed all the passengers they have collected?

> Hello BDD/passenger, what do you have to share today?

> I am noticing that you are guiding me to stay still/hide today...etc. I wonder why?

> It seems like you are worried about me today. What can I do differently? What do I need to watch out for or be aware of?

> There you are, [energy-giving passenger], where shall we go today?

Your client may need some support and guidance in picking up a few more life-affirming passengers to balance the noise, such as 'clarity, kindness' and 'connection' (values-guided passengers). Support them to be flexible with their journey and gentle with their bus; remind them to take it slowly. Support your client to plan and pack well (bringing all the processes of psychological flexibility with them) to keep themselves going when trying out a new route or exploring the passengers in a fresh way. Remind them to stop at times to take in the scenery and notice (and celebrate) how far they have come, and to consider where they want to go next.

Concluding Reflections

ACT facilitates an exploration and reframing of the ways of approaching the world through a focus on values and flexibility. ACT also invites an acceptance of even the difficult thoughts and experiences, including the experience of a distressing preoccupation with one's appearance: the experience of BDD.

There is often a drive to let go of or get rid of the things that have caused pain, loss and difficulty, but this in itself can create another layer of pressure. The letting-go of a way of living that may have been part of one's life for a long time can bring a sense of emotional dissonance. For example, many people who have experienced BDD yearn to work towards a happier and healthier life, but at the same time fear thinking that the difficult times have been for nothing. This is where the power of ACT can help soothe this dissonance and offer a space to live with all life's experiences. The real work and movement forward comes from holding all one's experiences with love and acceptance – seeing them as part of the journey and finding meaning and value in each and all of them.

Let us end with the metaphor of a garden to consider this powerful idea of acceptance. All gardeners know that some plants will try to take over all the space in the garden. These might be referred to as 'weeds'; yet these plants often have a place and a purpose. If we take the herb mint as an example, we note that it is medicinal, tasty and fragrant – but also, that it takes over if allowed. However, if mint is placed in a pot where its roots are contained it can provide its many benefits without taking over. Equally the stinging nettle and dandelion (more classic weeds) can also be used as food or fertiliser (and both make a delicious cup of tea!): a use can be found for them and they are of value. We can gain strength and knowledge from holding all experiences with love and acceptance. This facilitates a holding of the self with love and acceptance also.

References

Dehbaneh, M. A. (2019). Effectiveness of Acceptance and Commitment Therapy in improving interpersonal problems, quality of life, and worry in patients with body dysmorphic disorder. *Electronic Journal of General Medicine, 16*(1), em105.

Gillard, D., & Brown, F. J. (2016). *Acceptance and Commitment Therapy for dummies.* Wiley.

Harris, R. (2019). *ACT made simple: An easy-to-read primer on Acceptance and Commitment Therapy,* 2nd edn. New Harbinger Publications.

Hayes, S. C., Barnes-Holmes, D., & Roche, B. (2013). *Relational Frame Theory: A post-Skinnerian account of human language and cognition.* Plenum Publishers.

Hayes, S. C., Strosahl, K. D., & Wilson, K. G. (1999). *Acceptance and Commitment Therapy: An experiential approach to behavior change.* Guilford Publications.

Linde, J., Rück, C., Bjureberg, J., Ivanov, V. Z., Djurfeldt, D. R., & Ramnerö, J. (2015). Acceptance-based exposure therapy for body dysmorphic disorder: A pilot study. *Behavior Therapy, 46*(4), 423–431.

Pickard, A. J., Lumby, C., & Deane, F. P. (2021). True beauty lies within: Therapist interview of a client who received Acceptance and Commitment Therapy for body dysmorphic disorder. *Clinical Psychologist, 25*(2), 234–239.

Wilson, K. G., & DuFrene, T. (2008). *Mindfulness for two: An Acceptance and Commitment Therapy approach to mindfulness in psychotherapy.* New Harbinger Publications.

Chapter 11

Using the Compassionate Mind Approach with BDD

――――

ROSA HERNANDO HONTORIA

Introduction

The aim of this chapter is to offer a brief introduction to the use of the Compassionate Mind approach with body dysmorphic disorder (BDD). We will explore together:

- A basic understanding of Compassion Focused Therapy (CFT) and how we can use compassion to work with BDD.

- An alternative view of BDD as a self-critic and anxious part of the self that needs understanding and support.

- Some practical compassion skills and exercises to 'embody' and feel compassion rather than just 'saying compassionate things'.

I will not repeat the definition of BDD here as it has been stated previously in other chapters. I would, however, like to emphasise the role of shame in BDD. It would be fair to say that shame is the key emotion individuals with BDD experience. There may be different degrees of shame but every person with BDD feels ashamed of a specific feature or features of their appearance such as their nose, skin, shape of their face etc.

Paul Gilbert, a British psychologist, started developing CFT in the 1990s. While providing therapy to individuals using Cognitive Behaviour Therapy, he noticed that some of his clients would report that although they could logically see that, for example, they were not a failure or unlovable, they still *felt* that way. In particular, he noticed that the tone of voice they used to talk to themselves was very harsh. Paul Gilbert saw a need to help people to activate feelings of self-compassion to match their new self-compassionate thoughts. I often say to my clients that unless we feel and embody feelings of compassion when we practise self-compassionate talk, we might as well just be saying, 'fish and chips'!

A key process of Compassionate Mind Training (CMT) is the need to *feel* compassion rather than merely thinking compassionate thoughts; in other words, the need to 'embody' compassion.

CMT is a set of therapeutic skills which are utilised to help the person develop self-compassion for themselves and others and therefore, to, reduce feelings of shame. CMT is at the core of CFT. One of the key clinical presentations for which Gilbert wanted to use CFT was for feelings of shame. Needless to say, people who experience high levels of shame are very critical of themselves and lack self-compassion. Extreme and pervasive feelings of shame lead to overwhelming distress in people with BDD. Any therapist who has worked with BDD knows that an essential skill is for the person to develop a more compassionate relationship with themselves.

What Is Compassion?

It is important to emphasise the difference between the layperson's definition of compassion and the CFT definition. One of the challenges in teaching people to develop self-compassion relates to the word 'compassion' in itself. A lot of people have certain negative views of what 'compassion' means, including, for example, letting oneself off the hook or being weak and complacent.

From a CFT perspective, compassion is the sensitivity to the suffering of oneself and others with a commitment to try to alleviate and prevent it (Gilbert, 2010). From this perspective, there is a particular quality of compassion that is often overlooked and forgotten about. It is that of *courage*. A very simple but powerful way of thinking about self-compassion is viewing it as the commitment to do what is in our best interest even when this might be very difficult or scary.

Our brains are programmed to feel courage when we're being supported rather than criticised. This is because criticism tends to be perceived as a threat by the brain, while being supported helps us to feel safe. It is easier to feel courage to challenge ourselves from a place of safety rather than from a place of threat.

CFT highlights some ideas in relation to our common humanity:

- We all find ourselves in this life which throws challenges at us.

- We didn't choose our 'tricky brain'. Our minds have evolved in a way that makes them quite tricky and naturally vulnerable to getting caught up in unhelpful thinking-feeling loops (Irons & Beaumont, 2017).

- We didn't choose our genes, family, culture, time in history etc. (in this respect different times in history have valued different body shapes; we live in an era of extreme attention to physical appearance).

Therefore, the key message from CFT is: it is not our fault that we have emotional difficulties as we did not choose them, but it is our responsibility to learn how to manage them. This is an empowering message. It absolves us from blame and criticism for having difficult emotions but reminds us that we are the only ones who can be responsible for learning how to manage our tricky minds.

Understanding the Brain's Way of Regulating Emotions

One of the most helpful ways of understanding emotional regulation I have come across is the three-circles model we use in CFT. This model is illustrated in the diagram below.

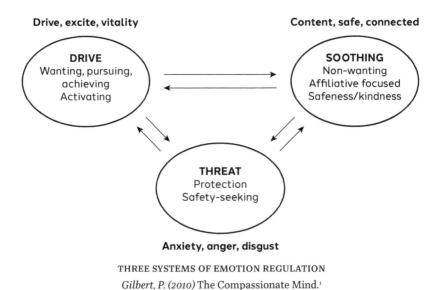

THREE SYSTEMS OF EMOTION REGULATION
Gilbert, P. (2010) The Compassionate Mind.[1]

---

1   Adapted and reproduced with permission of the Licensor through PLSclear.

I want to emphasise that this diagram is not simply a psychological theory but an illustration of real emotional and biochemical processes that take place in the brain.

The threat system is linked to emotions of anger, fear and disgust. It is designed to help us detect and respond to threats in our lives. It is worth noting that some people with BDD report feeling disgusted about the aspect of their appearance they are worried about. The threat system cannot tell the difference between a threat to our physical self, such as a lorry coming towards us, and a threat to our psychological self or identity, such as the fear of a body part being seen by another person as ugly.

It is also really helpful to distinguish between external threats and internal threats. Humans are very good at activating our threat systems, for example by criticising ourselves or catastrophising about bad things happening even when externally there are no threats at all.

Most people with BDD have clear negative images of how they think they look and attach negative meanings to this such as *People will judge me/humiliate me* and *I'm unlovable/worthless*. They are also extremely self-critical. In sum, they're experts at activating their threat system.

The function of the drive system is to give us positive feelings which guide us to seek out resources that will be helpful for us to survive and prosper (Gilbert, 2010). The soothing system, on the other hand, is activated when we feel safe and relaxed and are having positive and caring interactions with others and with ourselves.

We need all of these systems to survive and, ideally, they would be balanced; but often they are not. The threat system is the one which is most easily activated by default as it deals with 'urgent' threats. The threat and the drive systems tend to have a bit of a tricky relationship between them. This means that we often arrive into the drive system via the threat system. For instance, we might get the motivation to finish a project out of fear of missing the deadline and getting into trouble with our boss.

People with BDD engage in a lot of avoidant and safety behaviours in an attempt to 'fix the problem' (drive system) but unfortunately these strategies stem from the threat system and feed into the BDD and keep it going. Basically, the more time and mental energy the person invests into trying to solve the problem in this way, the more their brain gets the message that there's real danger. This validates to the brain that there's a serious problem and in turn this activates the threat system further. Thus, the solution becomes the problem. This is illustrated in the following diagram:

Need to move around the three circles system anti-clockwise to arrive into the drive system via the soothing system

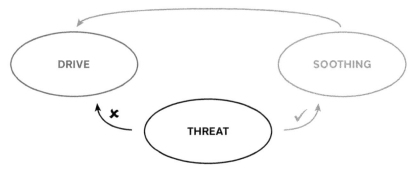

THE SOLUTION BECOMES THE PROBLEM
Gilbert, P. (2010) The Compassionate Mind.[2]

If we give a voice to the threat system as if it is communicating to the drive system, it might say something like (communicated in a harsh tone of voice):

> You are not good enough, so you better avoid certain situations where you might be judged. You must spend hours hiding/camouflaging your 'defect' and also constantly avoiding or checking in the mirror. You should also have cosmetic surgery. You must put as much energy as you can into correcting your defect. This must be your priority above everything else in your life.

This is using the drive system in an unhelpful way: arriving at 'drive' from 'threat'.

If we give a voice to the soothing system as if it is communicating to the drive system, it might sound something like:

> It's completely understandable that you feel anxious about being judged (given early experiences of bullying, feeling not good enough etc.). I'm really sorry you feel this way. It must be really tough for you. I really care about you and I'm here for you. I'm totally devoted to supporting you. I want to help you to invest your energy in dealing with your fears in a constructive way. Instead of engaging in your avoidant and safety behaviours, let's make a plan of positive things you can do to live your life in line with your values.

---

2   Adapted and reproduced with permission of the Licensor through PLSclear.

In this case, the energy in the drive system would be positive and constructive, in line with values-led goals.

Ultimately, the aim is to help the brain make a new link so that when the person has a BDD-related thought, they can respond from the soothing system rather than from the threat system. For example: *Ah, there's my anxious self telling me I'm ugly when I compare myself with that attractive person. I know this comes from a part of me that feels bad and unworthy. I don't need to pay attention to the content of the thoughts, and instead I am just going to direct my caring feelings towards that part of me whose sensitivity to these triggers stems from difficult past experiences.*

It is very important to highlight that the exercises I describe in this chapter are not to be taken as relaxation techniques to get rid of anxiety. They should rather be seen as practices that aim to activate the soothing system in the brain in order to connect with the courage needed to challenge the avoidant and safety behaviours that maintain the BDD.

Having described some of the basic theoretical ideas that underpin the use of self-compassion skills for working with BDD, I will now describe a number of practical skills for using embodied approaches from this perspective.

Basic Building Blocks for Compassion Practices
Imagery Skills
One of the most fascinating facts about the brain is that it cannot tell the difference between an image of something and the real thing. For example, if we imagine eating a lemon we might notice increased salivation, the same physiological reaction that would occur if we were eating a lemon in real life. This fact leads to good and bad news: if we imagine positive things, we feel good, but if we imagine negative things, we activate our threat system.

Most people with BDD have clear negative images of how they look so they are experts at activating their threat system. This, together with the fact that the brain can't tell the difference between physical and psychological threat, can make it very tricky to manage the brain. If, for example, we think/imagine someone is going to judge, humiliate or reject us, the brain believes it's true and if the level of the emotion is intense enough, it feels as if we might die! CFT recognises the power of imagery; therefore, this is one of the key skills used in a lot of the practices. Recent scientific findings have found that imagery has a bigger impact on our emotions than words alone, and that certain types of soothing imagery practices are linked to lower levels of stress hormones (Irons & Beaumont, 2017). Imagery is therefore a powerful way of activating our soothing system in the brain and, therefore, a key tool in some of the practices presented in this section.

Another important skill for practising compassion is being able to communicate it verbally. Below is a list of some of the key qualities of compassion with sentence stems of how we may communicate them:

- *Empathy*: It's understandable you feel that way – this is hard.

- *Sympathy*: I'm so sorry you are having a hard time.

- *Support*: I'm here for you and I'll help you find ways to overcome this and grow.

- *Courage*: By challenging yourself little and often you can grow and overcome your limitations.

- *Praise*: Focus on achievements, even if small – not failures. Praise yourself for your desire and effort to change.

- *Encouragement*: There will be blocks along the way but if you persevere it will get easier.

- *Distress tolerance*: This is really hard, but it will pass. When you commit to supporting yourself there are lots of tools you can learn to soothe yourself.

Basic Grounding Practice

For most of the exercises described in this chapter it is helpful to begin with a basic grounding practice to help clear the mind, focus and be present in the practice about to be undertaken. There are hundreds of versions of grounding practices and the one I am presenting here is just a basic version I often use with clients.

Find a time to be quiet and undisturbed. Start by sitting comfortably with both feet flat on the floor. During this practice it is highly likely that, sooner or later, the mind will wander away from the practice and get distracted with other things. This is totally normal; it is what minds do – they wander – so try not to get frustrated if this happens. Gently and patiently bring the mind back to the practice each time it wanders.

Next, bring your attention to the sensation of touch of the feet in contact with the floor. You could imagine you are like a tree with roots growing out of your feet deep into the ground, grounding you solidly, in this moment, in this place. Nothing else matters now, just observing your experience moment by moment.

Next, move your attention to the sensation of pressure of your body against the chair, allowing your weight to go down onto the chair, letting go of any tension and fully allowing the chair to hold you. Slow your breathing down gently without forcing it, breathing all the way down to the abdomen. Find a pattern of breathing that feels soothing for you.

The Compassionate Self Practice (Kolts et al., 2018)

This is one of the most basic and helpful practices we can use to activate our compassionate self. It is particularly helpful when we use multiple selves (described below) and is a way to embody compassion before we give a voice to the compassionate self, so the words match the feeling.

The essence of this practice is to imagine ourselves being compassionate towards someone we really care about like a best friend who is struggling. This practice takes around ten minutes. We want to ensure we will not be interrupted. It is really important to slow down and take our time to do this so we can fully engage with the details and make it more vivid and therefore more effective. We might want to play some relaxing music.

Start with the basic grounding practice described above.

Imagine you are sitting in front of a loved one who is struggling. Perhaps they are upset about some difficulty in their lives. It might help to remember a real time when this person was suffering or to imagine a hypothetical situation in which they would be suffering such as losing a beloved pet or going through a relationship break-up. Next, connect with the intention of being fully present for them. Connect with a wish to devote all your attention to this person, to be fully sensitive to their suffering, wanting to thoroughly understand what they are going through and connecting with your deepest commitment to try to alleviate their suffering.

You may want to adopt an upright body posture (you probably would not want to be slouching on the chair) but with a certain softness and free of tension, gently letting the shoulders drop. You may also want to slow down your breathing, gently, without forcing it, breathing all the way down to the abdomen. If the mind wanders, gently bring it back. Adopt a warm and soft facial expression and have a soft gaze in your eyes. You might want to imagine you have a soft and warm inner, compassionate smile. You may also want to use a warm tone of voice and speak at a slow pace. You could imagine saying something like 'I'm here for you', with a soft and warm tone.

Multiple Selves Practice

The Multiple Selves framework guides us to become aware of different parts of ourselves, viewing them as a separate person each with a set of thoughts, feelings, body sensations, memories etc. (Irons & Beaumont, 2017).

The basic idea is that we attach the identity of a separate person to a negative emotion. For example, instead of 'I am anxious', we might say 'My anxious self has been activated'. In doing so we create some distance from that emotion, thus gaining more objectivity and perspective. We then free up some space to embody another part of us that is courageous, wise and compassionate.

We can use multiple selves to work with any difficult emotion such as anger, fear, sadness etc. We start by identifying all of the components of the 'struggling self' such as 'angry', 'afraid' or 'sad'. We then activate our compassionate self and respond to the struggling self. For this, it is helpful to imagine that this self is someone we love and care about such as a relative or a dear friend. If someone we care about was struggling with a certain situation or problem and we wanted to support them, we would want to first understand how they are feeling, what their thoughts are about the situation, what it is reminding them of etc. We will now explore this in more detail.

Anxious Self or Critical Self?

In BDD, the anxious self is the same as the critical self: when the anxious self feels scared of being criticised or judged by others, it focuses on the perceived appearance 'defect' and warns the person to be very careful to try to avoid being judged.

An important part of the journey of recovery is to support your client to develop compassion for their BDD. This includes moving away from viewing BDD as a bully, but rather viewing it as a part of the self that is absolutely terrified of being judged, rejected and humiliated.

This part has probably endured extreme suffering for a very long time, feeling really bad and not good enough, worthless etc. It has probably had negative and/or traumatic experiences of being bullied, criticised or humiliated. Or perhaps it has grown up with a lot of praise about their appearance while simultaneously not feeling good enough as a person: therefore it has fused *looking* good with *being* good enough and worthy. It has developed lots of strategies and safety behaviours to try to keep the person safe (safety behaviours, avoidance, attention on the threat etc.).

It might be quite a novel idea for your client to develop compassion for their BDD rather than seeing it as a bully. Viewing BDD as a bully is an approach which is sometimes used in therapy and it has its merits; but it would interfere with having compassion for the BDD as it is very difficult to have compassion for a bully!

When we use the Multiple Selves model it is helpful to be systematic about it so we can keep on track and do it thoroughly in order to pay attention to all the different aspects. We begin by supporting our client to number and identify all the components of the anxious/critical self. It is helpful to prompt your client to choose a specific situation that is or has been a trigger. I will use first person perspective here as if the person with BDD/anxious self was speaking.

ANXIOUS SELF ABOUT GOING TO THE PARTY WHEN I THINK MY SKIN LOOKS BAD WITH BLEMISHES OR SPOTS

1. *Thoughts*: What thoughts might the anxious self have about this situation? If it could speak, what would it say?

    - My skin looks really bad today and I don't think I can go to the party.

    - If I go, people will notice my skin and feel sorry for me and think I'm inferior.

    - People don't value me as a person, so I need to at least be perfect in my physical appearance to be respected.

    - The other people will gossip about it and laugh at me.

    - Maybe if I spend two hours applying make-up to camouflage my skin I can go to the party as long as I don't talk to people for too long and avoid bright lighting areas.

2. *Body*: How does the anxious self feel in the body (e.g. muscle tension, tightness in chest area)?

   – Feel nauseous just thinking about it.

   – Feel tension in my chest and my head.

   – Heart beating faster.

3. *Behaviour*: If the anxious self was not worried about consequences, what would it really want to do? What does it really feel like doing?

   – Either avoid going to the party and stay at home feeling miserable. Or spend hours camouflaging and mirror checking, then going to the party but talking to people only briefly and frequent visits to bathroom to mirror check, avoiding areas with bright light etc.

4. *Function*: What is your anxious self trying to achieve?

   This is an extremely important aspect to identify and understand. The basic idea is that all negative emotions serve a protective function even when on the surface they just feel unhelpful and painful. Anxiety is the brain's way of warning us of danger and keeping us alive.

   So, in this example, the function of the anxious self might be:

   – To warn me that it is risky to go to the party; that something might happen to upset me, to make me feel rejected etc.

5. *Unintended consequences*: What is happening in the long term because of this person engaging in lots of avoidant and safety behaviours, such as spending a lot of time checking their skin in the mirror and avoiding social events?

   – Although the emotion of anxiety (or anxious self) aims to help and protect us, it's only focused on preventing danger in the moment/short term but it tends to backfire in the long term.

   – Paying too much attention to my skin and looking at it with a 'magnifying glass' approach makes me lose perspective. In the moment/short term if feels as if it's urgent that I do this but in the long term it backfires as I'm repeatedly teaching my brain that there is a threat.

- As I look at my skin searching for small flaws, the underlying message to my brain is that this is a dangerous problem and a threat. Thus, my brain will respond by raising the alarm in the form of anxiety every time I think about my skin/think about going to a party.

- If I avoid going to the party, I will miss out on socialising again and it will eventually affect my friendships as I keep avoiding social situations because of my BDD. I will stay at home ruminating which will make me feel depressed.

6. *Memories*: When feeling anxious about going to the party, what memories come to mind? This could be a memory of a similar trigger from the past such as:

- Being teased and bullied in school about my acne. It was so awful I have to avoid a repeat of this at all costs.

- A memory of the feeling of not feeling good enough.

- Getting lower grades than my best friend in school.

7. *Goal/need*: What would the anxious self want to feel at ease?

- To have perfect skin, to be 100 per cent sure that no one will judge me negatively.

- My anxious self wants to feel safe, accepted and valued. It wants not to feel the need to be perfect and so focused on physical appearance in order to feel worthy.

Once we have identified and understood these components of the anxious self, we move on to addressing them from the compassionate self. In this case, however, we want to switch the order of the first two so that the body/physiology becomes number one and the thoughts become number two. This is because before 'giving a voice' to the compassionate self to respond to the anxious self we want to *embody* compassion rather than communicating compassionate messages while feeling anxious in the body. Otherwise, we could be saying 'the right compassionate thing' but it would be just words. To put it simply, we want the words to match the emotion.

COMPASSIONATE SELF ABOUT GOING TO THE PARTY WHEN I THINK MY SKIN LOOKS BAD WITH BLEMISHES OR SPOTS

1. *Body/physiology*: After a simple grounding practice such as the one outlined towards the beginning of this chapter, your client will hopefully feel calmer and more relaxed and ready to speak from their compassionate self in the next step while feeling their words.

2. *Thoughts/message* from the compassionate self to the anxious self. *What would I say to a loved one in this situation?* It is really important in BDD not to engage with the content of the thoughts. We want to avoid saying things like 'Your skin is fine, I can't see any spots or your spots are hardly visible'; rather, communicate compassionate support by saying something like:

   > It is totally understandable that you are anxious about socialising and worried about being judged and humiliated given some of your early experiences. I am really sad that this is so difficult for you and that it causes you so much distress. I want you to know that I am here for you to support you and help you overcome these difficulties. Let's work on this together. You are not alone. I know it is difficult for you to believe this now, but I know that if you challenge yourself and step out of your comfort zone on a regular basis you will make progress. Remember the times when you have done this and felt better for it. I will also support you in learning tools to overcome your fears.

   Notice that in the supportive message above, there is no mention of the content of the fear, in this case facial skin. Also, I want to reiterate once more that the emphasis is on the feeling behind the words, not the words per se, and that it is absolutely key to imagine/practise saying the words with a warm and soft tone.

3. *Behaviour*: What would the compassionate self suggest to the anxious self to do in this situation? We want this behaviour to encompass the qualities of courage and wisdom.

   - We know that an absolutely key skill in overcoming BDD is attention training in order to practise focusing attention away from the preoccupation about physical appearance and outwardly towards the task at hand.

This might be a message about what to do:

> I know it is very difficult for you to stop but you know that the more you check your skin in the mirror the more anxious you will become. Try to focus your attention on thinking about the friends you will see at the party and how nice it will be to catch up with them. Even if you aim to only be there for a while, that will be a victory. You can use one of the grounding practices you have tried before you leave, to shift your attention away from your worries. I, the compassionate self, will go with you to the party and gently remind you to focus your attention outwardly.
>
> Remember to resist the urge to go to the bathroom to check your skin while you are there at the party. When you come back, praise yourself for having had the courage to go, add it to your list of victories and remind yourself that by continuing to challenge yourself you will definitely make progress.

4. *Function*: What is the compassionate self trying to achieve?

   – The compassionate self is always trying to get us to grow out of our limitations and to become the best version of ourselves.

5. *Unintended consequences*: Are there any negative consequences in the long term?

   – Good news here! There are never any negative consequences of acting from our compassionate self.

6. *Memories*: Do any memories come to mind when thinking of communicating compassion?

   – Remember: the memory does not need to match the 'theme' of the problem situation. It is the memory of the feeling that is important, i.e. feeling cared for, loved and supported when we were struggling.

7. *Goal/want (directly related to the function)*: The goal of the compassionate self is always to support us and help us to grow and overcome our limitations so that we can become the best version of our unique selves.

One word of warning here is that it is important to set time aside to do this exercise slowly, really devoting time to it. I would also suggest writing it all down, as writing forces us to slow down and really think about it. It is tempting to take a short cut and do it quickly in your mind but it tends to be less effective.

Given the role of developmental trauma in the development of BDD as we read about in Chapter 2, one of the most helpful ways in which compassion therapy can be used in working with BDD is by helping the person to cultivate compassion for their 'child self'. There are many practices that can facilitate this: I will just offer one example here. A key text with lots of ideas of how to work with the inner child is *Homecoming: Reclaiming and Championing Your Inner Child* (Bradshaw, 1991).

Using an Image of You as a Child to Soothe the BDD/Anxious Self

Ask your client to imagine they could travel back in time and meet with their 'child self', helping them to feel valued and loved and good about themselves. Prompt them to imagine how special this 'child self' is to them: how they believe in them and will always be there for them, supporting them.

When we move through imagery practices, it tends to be helpful to try to make the sense of the image as vivid as possible. We can do this by bringing a lot of detail to the image and also linking the details to all the senses such as sights, sounds, smells and touch. Some people are able to create more visual images than others, but it is important not to try to achieve a polaroid type image and instead focus more on the feelings generated by the image and the sense of the connection.

Your client may look at a photo of their younger self to help them connect more strongly with the details, or may simply imagine an image of their child self in their mind, as you prompt them with the following:

Look at the visual details such as the clothes they are wearing, their hair, any childlike features that may help activate feeling protective towards them like their little hands and fingers etc. Perhaps imagine what it would feel like if you were sitting them on your lap and cuddling them, noticing the warmth of their little body next to yours. Imagine gently and tenderly stroking their head or little hand and the soft touch of their skin.

Imagine the child is feeling sad or worried about some difficulty, possibly related to their BDD, and that you are comforting them about it. You can imagine telling them some supporting messages. The focus is not on the words but rather on you feeling caring, protective and supportive of them. In fact, sometimes the less we say the easier it will be to connect with the feelings so maybe try just saying something like 'It's okay, I'm here for you.' Do a gentle scan of your body and see if you can notice any specific physical sensations that are a sign of your caring system being activated in your brain, and relevant brain chemicals being released. This may take some practice, but examples of sensations people report are: a loosening of tension in the chest area, a spontaneous sigh, the body taking a deep slow breath on its own accord without conscious effort, and the shoulders dropping and tension leaving the muscles.

Soothing Imagery: The Perfect Nurturer (Lee, 2005)

What if we could create a figure that existed only for us and was 100 per cent devoted to supporting us when we are struggling: to praise us when we do well; to help us learn from our mistakes and encourage us when we fail; to help us to forgive ourselves when we make mistakes; to give us courage when we feel weak and afraid; to help us grow out of our limitations; to help us get up when we fall and get back on track; to support us in overcoming our fears, realising our full potential and becoming the best version of ourselves? What if we could create a sense of this figure in a way that felt real – if we could see every detail about them, hear the sound of their voice, and notice them carrying a scent of lavender or any other aroma we find soothing? What if we could feel their soft, warm, reassuring touch, even taste a food or drink they gave us? What if we could feel their presence as if they were really there, and truly feel the courage they want to instil in us?

What if by practising connecting with such a figure regularly in our minds, we could train our brains to develop an increasing sense of them and develop neural pathways that increased a sense of emotional safety in the presence of such a figure? It would then be easy to call up on them in our minds when we needed them and embody all those wonderful qualities listed above.

Would that not be amazing?

Well, guess what? *We can.*

As always with any soothing imagery it is helpful to start by using the basic grounding practice before leading your client in the following:

Allow your mind to think of a safe place. This could be a real place you know, or it might be an imaginary place. It might be indoors or outdoors, perhaps somewhere in nature like a garden, beach or mountains. Whatever it is, the only requirement is that this place represents safety, and you feel totally safe in it.

Now, connect with this place using all your senses; start by connecting with it visually. Look around and notice objects, colours, shapes etc. Connect also with sounds. What kind of soothing sounds can you hear in your safe place? It might be gentle singing of birds, the calming sound of a stream, maybe the sound of leaves gently rustling in a breeze. You might also like to include some soothing and calming scents in your safe place: perhaps the smell of your favourite flower or lavender. Finally, connect with a sense of touch: perhaps the warmth of the sun on your skin or choosing to touch some objects in your safe place. Connect with the texture, such as the feel of stroking a beloved pet, or the warm and soft white sand on a beach, or the feel of a stone. Know that this place welcomes you and wants you to be there. It exists only for you and only feels complete when you are there. It has been waiting for you to arrive.

Allow the image of a compassionate figure to appear in the distance. This figure might be a human being, someone you know or someone that you know of, like a figure from history or a book or film character that represents compassion. It could also be an animal or an element of nature like a tree, the ocean or a mountain or even just a light. The only requirement is that whatever it is, it can take on human qualities: the qualities of compassion. It has infinite empathy for your distress and difficulties, infinite understanding, infinite sympathy. This figure feels sad if you are sad, wants you to never feel alone with your difficulties. This figure also only exists for you and has been waiting for you to make contact with it. It is totally devoted to you and your wellbeing and wants to support you and help you in any way that you might need.

This compassionate figure wants you to grow and become the best version of yourself. It is totally devoted to helping you work through any obstacles that you might encounter in life. It also possesses an infinite courage that it wants to share with you. It also has infinite wisdom to know exactly what you're feeling in any moment and what might be a constructive path out of a challenge. It knows you better than anyone else in the world, even better than yourself. It knows the path you've been on in your life, so it knows that anything that you feel makes sense given this path. It knows that none of your difficulties are your fault. It wants you to develop the strength and courage to face any obstacles you might encounter.

Again, allow yourself to connect with this figure with all your senses. What would you like your ideal compassionate figure to look like or sound like? Would you like it to have any soothing scent? Would you like to make physical contact with it, perhaps by gentle touch or being embraced by it? Know that this figure is always available to you, willing to support you day and night. Whenever you're having a moment of difficulty, you can make contact with it.

Prepare yourself to say goodbye for now. Bring your attention back to the room you are in and the sensation of touch with the chair, floor or bed, noticing your breath.

Potential Obstacles to Using Self-Compassion Practices with BDD

It is very common to meet some resistance when we suggest the use of self-compassion skills to clients experiencing BDD. There are a number of reasons for this.

As mentioned earlier, some clients (and people generally) have negative beliefs about compassion. Some people view self-compassion as a weakness and letting ourselves off the hook. In reality, self-compassion involves facing our difficulties and moving towards difficult emotions as well as the motivation and commitment to change ourselves. This requires courage and strength (Welford, 2012). It can be helpful to point out that key historical figures who represented compassion were far from weak such as Mahatma Gandhi and Nelson Mandela.

It is also not uncommon for people to believe or feel that they do not deserve compassion. In these cases, it can be helpful for them to ask someone they trust what they think about this (Welford, 2012), asking themselves if they would feel the same way about someone else in the same situation.

Another common obstacle, related specifically to suggesting exercises that involve working with the 'child self', is that some clients might have negative feelings about their younger self. For example, they might blame themselves as a child thinking things like *I should have been brighter, stronger, less greedy with food (if being overweight led to bullying), more interesting (if it was difficult to make friends)* etc. In these cases, it is necessary to first help the person to develop compassion for their younger self. Children lack the capacity to take responsibility for themselves and they need the guidance and support of responsible parents/carers to help them overcome any difficulties or limitations. It is never realistic to expect a young child to overcome challenges on their own. It is an intrinsic principle of the lifecycle that children need protection and guidance from adults. This obstacle, however, can be quite entrenched and difficult to overcome. Therefore using other practices outside of those related to the 'child self' in the early stages of therapy may be more supportive for some clients.

Concluding Reflections

When I came across Compassion Focused Therapy, I simply fell in love with it and have been passionate about it since. I find it offers tremendous possibilities for transforming longstanding and entrenched negative emotions, particularly those linked to self-criticism, which typically leads to unimaginable suffering for people with BDD. There is of course much more to say and much more work that can be done in using the principles I have described here. Yet I hope I have been able to provide enough of an introduction to demonstrate the enormous potential self-compassion can have in the context of BDD.

References

Bradshaw, J. (1991). *Homecoming: Reclaiming and championing your inner child.* Judy Piatkus Ltd.

Gilbert, P. (2010). *The Compassionate Mind.* Constable and Robinson Ltd.

Irons, C., & Beaumont, E. (2017). *The compassionate mind workbook.* Little, Brown Book Group.

Kolts, R. L., Bell, T., Bennett-Levy, J., & Irons, C. (2018). *Experiencing Compassion-Focused Therapy from the inside out.* The Guilford Press.

Lee, D. A. (2005). The perfect nurturer: A model to develop a compassionate mind within the context of cognitive therapy. In P. Gilbert (ed.), *Compassion: Conceptualisations, research and use in psychotherapy* (pp. 326–351). Routledge.

Welford, M. (2012). *Building your self-confidence using Compassion Focused Therapy.* Constable and Robinson Ltd.

Chapter 12

Eye Movement Desensitisation and Reprocessing for BDD

——————

BEVERLEY HUTTON

I have been running the Reading Body Dysmorphic Disorder (BDD) Foundation support group since 2016 and, since that time, have worked with increasingly more people with BDD, offering primarily Eye Movement Desensitisation and Reprocessing therapy (EMDR) since 2019. EMDR has been a dramatic experience for some, and it is a privilege to share something of those experiences here, with very grateful thanks to those who have allowed me to share their stories with you.

I initially started seeing Charlene (name changed for confidentiality purposes) for psychodynamic psychotherapy before we decided to try EMDR. She was my first EMDR BDD client, and it was to be an astonishing experience for both of us. She puts it into her own words:

> I have suffered from BDD for approximately 17 years. I really wasn't enjoying life and it felt as if I was just existing and had no future. After six months of EMDR I was shocked by how much I had improved. To be able to wake up not feeling dreadful or anxious about looking in the mirror was unbelievable. I now have the relationship with my mum that I longed for, and never thought would be possible. I never feel lonely or empty anymore and I have discovered a newfound confidence in my little soul!

During sessions, Charlene regularly went back to remembering childhood toys, and even being in the pram. She was able to process various early traumatic events that up until then had been too difficult for her to access and work on.

This has largely been my experience of EMDR since. EMDR enables people to get behind the powerful distraction of the BDD symptoms to work on the root of the difficulties. This chapter will explain how it manages to do that through looking back over the work with another client, Sophie (name also changed for confidentiality purposes).

What is EMDR?

EMDR was discovered by accident in 1987 by Francine Shapiro (1948–2019), an American psychologist, who happened to notice that when she was looking from side to side while out walking one day, disturbance from negative thoughts and memories disappeared without conscious effort. When she tried to think about the same things again, they were neither as upsetting nor as vivid as they were before. Francine set out to experiment further, going on to eventually develop a standard protocol that is now used internationally in the treatment of a wide range of mental health symptoms, though is most widely known for its successful treatment of PTSD (post-traumatic stress disorder).

To understand how EMDR works, it is helpful to first understand what happens when you are traumatised. If you experience an over-whelming single traumatic event or are exposed to repeated distress over a prolonged period of time, your natural abilities to cope can become overloaded. All the associated disturbing content can then remain in the amygdala part of your brain where it continues to get activated by other similar emotions and events in the present. Memories are stored not only as visual images, but also as physical and sensory sensations, emotions and thoughts. They can be triggered by a similar reminder, for example a familiar smell, which sends you back to the original traumatic experience.

Even if the memory itself is long forgotten, the painful feelings such as anxiety, terror, anger or despair can continue to be triggered in the present. EMDR helps us to reach the associated connections within our memory networks which enable the brain to process the original traumatic memory. Every time a person is triggered by something in the present, it's because it's connected to something similar from the past held within the nervous system. The response however can feel completely outside of the person's control, and manifest in experiences such as flashbacks and panic attacks.

When we use EMDR to process the event or fear, the associated content starts to shift from the amygdala to the hippocampus where it can then be stored safely as having happened in the past, without causing further present-moment triggering.

BDD is a powerful coping mechanism that distracts the brain from thinking about difficult experiences from the past that may have triggered the onset of BDD. Regardless of what caused the BDD originally, it is the BDD symptoms that cause significant distress in a person's current experience and for which they seek help. Whilst we can focus on those symptoms initially, as processing continues, the focus is more likely to be around the other events that may have been repressed. As a coping strategy, BDD is highly successful. Instead of focusing on the distressing events that caused the onset of symptoms, the person becomes preoccupied instead with an aspect of their body and, as a distraction, turns this into something to be feared and hated. As the obsession with the distorted perspective becomes increasingly distressing, the more the original experience(s) are pushed out of mind and 'forgotten'.

EMDR enables us to work on repressed content alongside the BDD symptoms without the person becoming overly distressed. It is a gentle and safe procedure, as you will see from some of the work Sophie undertook in her sessions.

What Happens in an EMDR Session?

Eye movements, similar to those during REM sleep, are recreated simply by asking the client to watch something moving backwards and forwards across their visual field. Hand-held pulsators and headphones can be used for additional stimulation, and for online sessions, bilateral butterfly tapping[1] with closed eyes can be used. The eye movements last for short sets before the client is asked to report back on whatever was noticed during each set. The client may notice changes in thought, visual images, physical sensations and emotions. With repeated sets, the memory tends to gradually lose intensity and may fade altogether.

When working on a distressing event or situation, we first need to find the point of the experience that causes the most disturbance. One way of doing this is to ask the client to imagine taking a still photo of the very worst part of the situation, and to ask what they would see in this image. This is called our 'Target', and it is the starting point from where we begin processing and to which we will repeatedly return to assess how we're doing. Bilateral stimulation (BLS) commences and as the

---

1   See Appendix B for more on butterfly tapping.

client progresses along a memory channel, emotions, images, physical sensations and thoughts will naturally surface until there is nothing left.

In EMDR, we use the analogy of looking out of a train window at the scenery passing by. If we see a tree, for example, we just want to notice it and not stop the train to get out and examine the tree in detail. Whether it's an image or a sensation, we just notice it and let it pass, because it's a stepping-stone to the next stone on the journey. Some people will find themselves jumping from one memory to another, but the brain can be trusted to go where it needs to go and bring to the surface what it needs to. As the memories and experiences come into conscious awareness, like drawers and files being opened, they quickly pass into the hippocampus for storage as a historical experience as the next file is opened.

At the end of each memory channel, we return to the Target to assess where we have got to. People will usually report a slight change, and maybe another emotion or thought will surface as they look at it. This is the start of the next channel. As each channel is cleared, we keep returning to the Target to check, until the person can say it no longer causes any distress. They may say that the Target has gone blurry, or they can't see it anymore, or it's transformed in some way, as you'll see later in the session transcripts.

Let's look now at what happened in a series of sessions with Sophie (all names and identifying details removed for confidentiality) so that you can understand the progression of her course with EMDR. Sophie is a young woman who has suffered with severe anxiety over her appearance since early childhood, which developed into BDD in her teenage years. Sophie's anxiety was directly caused by very cruel criticisms about her appearance at the hands of her mother. Sophie's mother was a dominating woman who seemed to project all of her insecurities about herself on to Sophie.

Therapy Session 1
Phase 1 (History Taking)
Understanding the background history forms part of this first phase of the eight phased protocol. The phases are broken up into History Taking, Client Preparation, Assessment, Desensitisation, Installation, Body Scan, Closure and Reassessment of Progress.

During this first phase we began by breaking down the disturbing memories related to Sophie's mother into the Earliest, Worst and more

Recent, starting first with the earliest difficult memory related to her mother. Sophie described a traumatic scene wherein her mother said Sophie was so disgusting she needed to scrub the disgust off her. She proceeded to manhandle her into the shower to roughly scrub off whatever it was she thought she was seeing and perceived as disgusting. This had been a terribly confusing and frightening experience for young Sophie who had no idea why she was so disgusting to her mother but, as young children tend to do, she believed what she was told by her primary caregiver.

Phase 2 (Client Preparation)

During the second phase, the process was explained to Sophie. She was asked to notice whatever came up and reminded that she was only processing old material and to trust her brain with where it took her. She was reminded that she would be able to stop the process at any time and that she was in control.

Phase 3 (Assessment)

We broke the memory down as follows.

The part of the memory which caused the most distress to Sophie was that of being scrubbed really hard by her mother, so this was the Target image. I asked Sophie to describe how this experience made her feel about herself, or how it defined her. This is the Negative Cognition (NC) or self-belief associated with the experience which was, *I am disgusting*, rather understandably. The associated emotions were embarrassment, shame, upset and anxiety. As Sophie had previously undertaken a lot of other therapy on this memory before, it only had a relatively low level of distress and so was quite a good first memory to work on to see how she got along with EMDR. The Subjective Unit of Distress Score (SUDS) is measured on a scale of 0–10 with 10 being the worst imaginable. Sophie scored the memory as a 3. Sophie was asked to notice where she was feeling any physical sensations in her body as we talked about the experience, and these were noted as being in her chest. Sophie was then asked to focus on the Target and the NC that 'she is disgusting' while BLS was applied using TouchPoints,[2] a device I have found very helpful for online work. (All our sessions were conducted on Zoom during the Covid pandemic lockdown.)

---

2   See Appendix B for more on TouchPoints.

Phase 4 (Desensitisation)

Sets of BLS will be shown by the symbol ✦. After each set, I asked Sophie, 'What do you notice now?' After she reported back, I usually replied with 'Just go with that' or 'Just notice'. This is important so as not to interfere with the processing. (I don't want to take Sophie off on a tangent with any interpretations because her brain knows where it needs to go.)

Sophie was asked to focus on the Target (being roughly scrubbed in the bath), alongside her NC of 'I'm disgusting' as we started the BLS. She was asked to notice anything at all that came up, whether an image, an emotion, thought or sensation, as it may have been important and linked. She was reminded that she was completely in control and could stop the process at any time if she wanted by raising her hand.

✦

B: What do you notice?
S: I can see her face and my own face, and the reactions.
B: Good, just go with that. ✦
S: I remember crying and how much it hurt where she was scrubbing. ✦

(After each answer, I encouraged Sophie to continue, with similar words such as 'Just notice', or to remind her that she is just an observer. I won't continue to include these responses below.)

S: I'm feeling ashamed and don't know what to do. ✦
S: I'm picturing the bathroom, remembering the sink and the tiles. ✦
S: I'm remembering the bathroom feeling cold, and I can smell the same familiar smell. ✦
S: I have got into my childhood bed to go to sleep. ✦
S: Just being in my bed is helping me to feel safe and calm. ✦
S: Thinking of the bed is making me feel sleepy. ✦
S: My brain feels quite calm, but my back feels sore, and my hands are tingling. ✦
S: I'm noticing a rumbling feeling of anger towards her now. ✦
S: I'm feeling even more angry now. ✦
S: I'm imagining myself fighting back. In reality, I was submissive and kind, and could never fight back because she was strong. ✦

At this point I asked Sophie if there was anybody who might be able to help her. Before the session we had installed not only a Safe Place, but also a Resource Team. These are characters that Sophie had chosen to help her if she got stuck in situations during the processing. Sophie had chosen three Nurturing and Compassion figures, three Protector figures and one Wisdom figure to choose between depending on the situation. The characters can be people Sophie knows, or they can be historical, mythological, from movies or books, faith-based or even animals. A pet cat or dog works really well as a Nurturing and Compassionate figure as the person can connect with the affection between them. This exercise, along with that for the Safe Place, can be found in Appendix B at the end of the book and can be used as a grounding exercise. Sophie had chosen the following for her Resource Team:

For Nurturing and Compassion:

- Toby, a pet dog.

- Nick, her brother.

- Jess, a friend.

For Protection:

- Finley, her fiancé.

- Sascha, a friend.

- Mr B (a movie character).

For Wisdom:

- Nick, her brother.

B: Is there anybody you could imagine bringing in to help you from your team?

S: Finley. ✤

S: I'm feeling a lot better because in my mind I can see that Finley has got her by the scruff of the neck and is saying, 'What are you doing?' I feel better because I was feeling defenceless. I couldn't fight back as a child. ✤

S: I feel more loved and protected. ✤

S: I can hear Finley's voice in my head telling me that she is a bully, rather than feeling any of the usual shame. ✤

S: My mind has jumped forwards to the present time. I have a sense of not being in that situation anymore. ✤

S: I'm just sitting on my sofa looking out of the window, and I'm feeling relaxed and happy. ✤

Once this channel was clear I asked Sophie to return to the Target to reassess and to notice whatever arose.

S: The image is similar, but the feelings aren't very strong. Previously it would instantly make me feel just as I did when I was a child but now it doesn't. ✛

B: If you were to rate the level of distress now, 0–10, what would it be?

Sophie reported that her level of distress was now a score of 1. Once we have the SUDS down to 0–1, we can move into the next phase and begin to work on installing a new Positive Cognition (PC) or self-belief to replace the NC 'I'm disgusting'.

Phase 5 (Installation)

Sophie felt that a more realistic self-belief/PC at this stage was, 'I'm normal'. I asked Sophie to think about the original memory and the words 'I'm normal' and to tell me how true this felt on a score of 1–7, with 7 being completely true. This Validity of Cognition (VOC) is tested after more repeated sets of BLS to strengthen it. Once Sophie felt that she was able to believe this without any other intrusive negative thoughts and could give it a score of 7, we moved into Phase 6.

Phase 6 (Body Scan)

Sophie was asked to close her eyes and concentrate on the incident and the PC while scanning her body from top to toe to check for any physical sensations anywhere. If there were any sensations, I would have asked her to focus on the physical symptom alongside the BLS until it cleared.

Phase 7 (Closure)

We concluded the session with an explanation and reminder that processing would continue after the session had finished over the next few days. I told Sophie that she may be aware of new material that surfaces, or that it might continue to surface at an unconscious level. Sophie was encouraged not to try to understand any processing but just to notice it, and maybe jot it down for the next session.

Phase 8 (Reassessment)

When Sophie returned for her next session, we checked whether any new material had surfaced and we reassessed how she scored the incident 0–10. If we hadn't managed to get the SUDS down to 0 by the end of the session, it may have dropped by the time we met again. If more material had surfaced, it may have gone up.

Therapy Session 2

In Session 2, we worked on the Worst memory related to Sophie's mother. This was a memory of her mother criticising her skin and looking at her intently with absolute disgust.

Phase 3

Target: My mother's face up close to mine inspecting my skin.

NC: 'I'm disgusting'.

Emotions: Upset, particularly about my skin.

SUDS: 8.

Body sensations: Back of throat.

Phase 4

Sophie started by focusing on the Target of her mother's face up close to hers, inspecting her skin alongside the NC of 'I'm disgusting'. ✤

S: I feel embarrassed and small. ✤
S: I'm focusing on my mother's face and I'm feeling scrutinised and picked apart. ✤
S: I feel ashamed, like it's my fault. ✤
S: I want to run away and hide. ✤
S: I'm hiding in my bedroom, and I don't know if it's now or then. [The person always has one foot in the present and one in the past, so the experiences can often feel as if they're happening in the present moment, particularly with physical sensations.] ✤
S: I spent most of the following years hiding in my bedroom. ✤
S: I'm 13 years old and I'm upstairs. I'm having an argument with my mother because she's cross that I'm spending too long getting ready, and I'm shouting at her, saying, 'I'm only doing this for you!' ✤
S: I remember crying and thinking that when my skin looks bad, I get into trouble, and when I spend too much time covering it up, I get into trouble as well. I feel hopeless. ✤

S: I'm aware of my brain trying to solve a problem but I don't know how to get out of this situation. ✢

S: Now I'm feeling angry again because if she hadn't said anything, I wouldn't be in this situation now. ✢

S: I'm thinking about somebody else I know with bad skin who doesn't try to cover it up. ✢

S: My brain is trying to work out how I feel about that person not covering up her skin. Part of me wants to be able to do that, but another part of me thinks it's disgusting. [Here we see some rational reasoning that will help Sophie as she compares it to her irrational thinking about herself.] ✢

S: I feel like I'm different. She may be able to go out with her skin like that, but I'm not allowed. It's not acceptable for me. ✢

S: It's now Christmas Day, after lunch, and everyone is having a nap except me. I've done all the washing up and have taken my make-up off. My mother wakes up and complains at me for having taken it off. ✢

S: I'm feeling annoyed because I've done all the washing up, which nobody has noticed. Unless I look good, I'm worthless. ✢

S: I'm back in my bedroom and I have to hide away. ✢

S: My bed is my safe place where I can be myself without anybody looking at me. ✢

S: I'd like to stay in my bed forever but another part of me is reminding me of lots of things saying, 'What about this?' and 'What about that?' It's reminding me of some nicer things. ✢

At this point I asked Sophie to imagine holding the option of staying in bed in one hand and all the nicer things in the other hand, and then to imagine looking between her hands in turn and to notice which felt like the strongest or best option. ✢

S: The bed option initially seemed like the best option, but as I continued to think about all the hard times, they began to feel less important. The other hand, however, was showing me all the nicer alternatives. It was like I was holding bubbles that represented these two options, and gradually the positive bubbles were getting bigger. ✢

S: I've got lots of positive things going on in my life now, and although there is some anxiety, there are also a lot of positive feelings. ✢

S: I'm thinking about Finley and all the things we're going to do together in the future. ✢

S: My mind is pulling me back to what I was thinking about before and the negative feelings are saying that I can't have that because I shouldn't be out there doing nice things. ✦

S: It's not super strong, but a little voice is saying, 'You don't deserve this. It's all going to fall apart.' ✦

At this point I thought it best not to proceed further without rescripting the scene on Christmas Day, so I asked Sophie to think about who she might need to help her and what she needed them to do.

S: I'm going to take Finley and Mr B with me to help me. ✦

S: They're standing between me and my mother, defending me and shouting at her, telling her how I've done all the washing up and she's not even allowing me to relax and take my make-up off. ✦

S: My mother looks shocked, then scared. Then she seemed to shrink. ✦

S: It's silly, but I imagined having a hug from Finley and Mr B. My mother was like a mouse running around on the floor squealing! ✦

S: My mother has a tail like a mouse and Mr B stood on her! ✦

S: I'm feeling much better. It's even comical. ✦

With Sophie now feeling a lot calmer and more positive, I asked her to return to the Target to have another look at it.

S: I can still see her coming close to my face, but I feel like an observer. ✦

S: I have this urge to push her away. Then I hugged myself just as I had felt the hug from Finley and Mr B in the previous scene. [The aim with using the Resource Team is to gradually help the client to develop the ability to be more compassionate towards themselves and be better equipped to resolve situations that arise. Some can use an adult version of themselves to help their younger self during processing as they develop a stronger compassionate and protective mindset.] ✦

S: I've now walked out of the room with my younger self. ✦

S: I feel more comforted. ✦

I asked Sophie to return to assess the Target again.

S: I was trying to see my mother's face, but now it all feels very blurry.

SUDS: 0–10? < 1. It doesn't feel anywhere near as emotional.

Phase 5

PC: 'I'm normal.'

VOC: 7.

Phase 6

Body Scan: I can feel my skin, as if it's bad. [We tapped on this along with the PC 'I'm normal' until the sensation reduced.]

Therapy Session 5

In this session we target Sophie's distress over her nose. We start by using a memory about her nose.

Phase 3

Target: Having a meal with my family and my mother making a joke about my nose. (Sophie describes the worst part of this memory as when she was in her room on her own afterwards thinking about it, when all of her feelings of fear of judgment arose within her.]

NC: 'I'm ugly.'

Emotions: Humiliation, shame.

SUDS: 5.

Location of body sensation: Throat and sternum.

Phase 4

As usual, Sophie starts by focusing on the Target and NC. ✤

S: I remember being in my room thinking about all the negative memories about my nose. ✤

S: I'm thinking about my brother's nose, which is a perfect, small nose. I've always wanted his nose. If he was a girl, he'd be prettier than me. He should have been the girl and me the guy. ✤

S: I'm feeling anxious. I still don't know what I look like because when I look in the mirror I see different versions of myself. ✤

S: I've gone back to going shopping and being in a changing room with mirrors at different angles. I saw my profile for the first time and felt paralysed with fear and horror. Part of that was my nose. Everything looked distorted and I had no idea how I would ever be able to leave that changing room. ✤

S: I'm feeling the fear about my mother's joke, and thinking that I am the joke, and everyone knows that I'm this ugly creature and they're just being polite about it. ✤

S: I'm still feeling fearful about the uncertainty of how I look and other people thinking bad things about me. ✢

S: My mind is trying to reassure me. I'm thinking back to other negative comments and I can't think of any except from my mother. ✢

S: I'm trying to remind myself that people still want to be my friend. I used to think that nobody wanted to be my friend when I was younger because of the way I looked. ✢

S: I went back to school where I'm feeling insecure because of some of the comments made. ✢

S: I'm having extreme memories from that time; of people telling me what was wrong with me. ✢

S: I'm in my bedroom at school and someone has said in front of the whole class that they feel sorry for me because I need a make-over, and I went to my room and cried. I didn't want to exist. ✢

S: [Sophie sighed] I felt really alone. I thought about ending it. [She continued crying.] ✢

S: We all had to wear ties with the uniform. I tied mine to the wardrobe and was pulling my head through it to hang myself when somebody came in, so I quickly took my head out so they couldn't see what I was doing. ✢

S: They asked me what I was doing, but I didn't say anything. They said they had heard that I was upset, and they tried to make me feel better. I said to myself at this point that if I don't improve the way I look within six months, I'd try again. ✢

S: [Sophie sighed and was crying again.] Why is this coming up now when it was so long ago? ✢

S: I have this sense of shame about being me. It's like a fundamental level of shame that I can't shift. ✢

S: I wish I had somebody by my side, helping me to navigate the world. ✢

B: Who would you like to invite in from your team?

S: I think I want them all there. ✢

S: I'm back in my bedroom at school, and everybody is there. Finley is giving me a hug. My brother and Jess are reassuring me. The others are there too. ✢

S: Finley and Nick are telling me how much they love me. ✢

S: It's almost like it's me trying to convince me that it's true. ✢

S: I'm feeling very wanted and loved, which is nice. [Sophie cried.] I know they'll protect me. ✢

B: Just connect and stay with that feeling of being loved and protected. ✢

S: I'm feeling okay to be me. ✢

S: I can see them walking alongside me, and I feel better. ✢

S: I feel lighter. ✢

B: Have another look at the Target now. What do you notice?

S: I have this fear of Finley waking up one day and realising that I'm actually gross. ✢

S: Half of my brain is trying to reassure me because we've been together so long and he doesn't react any differently to whether I've got make-up on or not, but the other half of me is thinking about looking like Gollum standing next to him in photos. ✢ [Notice the opposing arguments that are beginning to take shape.]

S: I'm feeling powerless, like I'm not in control. ✢

S: I just went blank but then I felt more relaxed, but I don't know why. ✢

S: I'm imagining getting hugs from Finley and feeling comforted.

B: Notice how that feels and register it. ✢

S: I went back to when my mother had made fun of me, and I told Finley how I felt. He was shocked and is reassuring me. ✢

S: I'm thinking about wanting a different nose, but also not wanting one at the same time. It feels the same as me not being able to work out what I look like. I would like a little nose, but it could go wrong, and I don't want to look like that. I'm debating it in my mind. ✢

S: Finley doesn't want me to do anything about my nose. He doesn't want me to change a single part of me. ✢

S: I'm suddenly feeling it's safe not to make any changes. ✢

S: I'm thinking that if I did get a nose job and then had children and my children had a different nose to me, how would that make them feel? ✢

S: Finley has a big nose, too, and I like his nose. That makes us similar. ✢

S: I'm thinking about the fact that Finley doesn't think about his nose and so nor should I.

I asked Sophie to return to the Target and assess it again.

S: I feel more detached from it.

SUDS: 0

Phase 5
PC: 'I'm fine as I am.'

VOC: 7.

Phase 6

Body Scan: Fine.

Therapy Session 7

In this session we're focusing on Sophie's distress over her skin. She uses a memory at school when she was 13 years old and had a spot on her face.

Phase 3

Target: A friend staring at a spot on my face in the classroom and the horror I felt.

NC: 'I'm disgusting.'

Emotions: Humiliation.

SUDS: 8.

Location of body sensation: Tummy and tightness across my chest and shoulders.

Phase 4

Sophie starts by focusing on the Target and the NC. ✤

S: I can see the classroom. ✤

S: I can see her staring at me. ✤

S: I'm not in control of my skin, which is so stressful and anxiety provoking. ✤

S: I'm feeling very angry and frustrated that I can't control my skin. ✤

S: I'm younger now. I remember crying. ✤

S: I've just jumped to the present time and I still feel like people are judging me for having bad skin or wearing too much make-up. I worry about that a lot. ✤

S: I'm feeling very upset. I feel like I'm still struggling with the same problems and worry that people will think I'm vain for wearing too much make-up and that I'm actually really ugly. ✤

S: I'm worrying that I'll never be normal. I'll never be able to be a mother. I'm really scared. [She started crying.] ✤

S: I'm thinking that people must be thinking I should be over this by now, and that my bad skin is my own fault. ✤

S: I'm back to feeling angry over my skin that I'm not able to control it. [Crying.] ✤

S: I don't know what to do. ✤

S: I'm aware of a fundamental feeling that my skin is not okay and it's not acceptable to be seen by others. But Finley will say that I look okay without make-up, but I feel confused because I'm not seeing what he sees and I don't know what is acceptable. ✤

S: I get the smallest spot and then even a colleague at work pointed it out from the other side of the room and laughed at me. ✤

S: I cried and felt so embarrassed. I went home and cut my hair into a fringe to cover it up. I can feel everyone looking at me. ✤

S: I can't change the fear that everyone is looking at me and I can't see what Finley is seeing. I feel paralysed. ✤

S: I want somebody to protect me, or to say that I'm okay.

B: Would you like to bring in somebody from your team?

S: Finley. ✤

We go back to rescript the original memory.

S: I can see her laughing at me and then Finley comes in. He's 6'2" and my friend is really small, and he shouted at her. Now he's giving me a big hug. ✤

S: Now, I've gone to the work memory. I can feel the memory more vividly. I can actually feel the spot on my face. The colleague is laughing at me. Finley grabs him by the collar and shoves him away and tells him to shut up. ✤

S: I've switched back to the original memory again and I remember going into the bathroom and crying. I'm bringing Finley in there to be with me. ✤

S: I'm focusing on Finley cuddling me in the bathroom as I wanted comfort then. ✤

S: I've gone back to the work memory. I go back to my desk and I've got Finley with me and I'm focusing on him telling me it's okay. ✤

S: I'm now thinking again about the time when I came home from school and was stuck upstairs unable to come out and I imagined Finley coming in and gently pulling me away from the mirror and talking to me. He's saying it's okay. ✤

S: He's holding my hand and we go downstairs together. I was worried about seeing my family without make-up, so he's taking me by the hand. ✤

S: I'm noticing that my tummy is rumbling, and I'm remembering that I wouldn't be able to have any food until I felt okay to be seen, which might take hours and hours. So, Finley is taking me downstairs to get some toast. [Sophie's tummy was actually rumbling a lot during this as she remembered not being able to eat. This is a body memory.] ✢

S: My mind is trying to sabotage things by remembering various things that my mother would say, but Finley is standing between me and her, shielding me so I can eat my toast. ✢

S: I was looking at my mother and thinking about how dominating she was, but then making her smaller and thinner and more frail. ✢

S: She's shrinking. I'm seeing her sat on her usual seat but she's shrinking along with the fear. ✢

S: She is now so small that she can't see over the table so she can't see me. ✢

S: Before I needed Finley there as a shield but now we're just laughing. I'm feeling more relaxed. ✢

S: It feels completely different now. ✢

Sophie assessed the Target again.

S: I can now see Finley there and my friend is scared of him.

SUDS: 0. 'I can't believe it!'

Phase 5
PC: 'I'm normal – all teenagers get spots.'

VOC: 7.

Phase 6
Body Scan: Fine.

Sophie continued to make really good progress. She was always amazed by how she felt by the end of the session about each of the scenarios we focused on. It is not uncommon for clients to experience a sense of disbelief and to question whether improvements can last after so many years of suffering with BDD.

Concluding Reflections
BDD is a developmental process usually starting in early childhood. In order to survive, a young child needs their environment to be safe, which is particularly difficult when there is a felt sense of unsafety in the family home. The child instinctively assumes that they are the cause of the

problem; that whatever is happening to and/or with their primary caregiver(s) must be because they are not good enough, not pretty enough, not the right gender etc. Children tend to take all of the blame and shame into themselves and, because of the level of their brain maturity, they may perceive these bad feelings as being related to their physical appearance. They may come to the faulty conclusion that if they could just fix the way they look, everything would be okay. A relentless search for a solution to fix the problem of their appearance then ensues, which fails to change how they feel inside as it was never their appearance that needed fixing in the first place.

Gradually, with the help of EMDR, the person can see for themselves how their brain has diverted them away from the distressing emotions and into their body. EMDR enables the person to make these important connections, with often astonishing and dramatic results. EMDR is fast becoming recognised as a very effective treatment for a wide range of mental health symptoms but there is very limited clinical research so far in the area of BDD due to lack of funding. I hope that this is something that will change over time because I have seen it make an enormous difference in my own work with BDD.

At the current time in the UK, EMDR is often only available on the NHS for the treatment of PTSD, so EMDR for BDD generally has to be on a private basis. Unlike other modalities, it is not necessary to find somebody who specialises in BDD with EMDR. You can find an EMDR therapist in your area by searching the EMDR Register: https://emdrassociation. org.uk/find-a-therapist

If you would like to see a recording of an EMDR session I undertook for a webinar for the BDD Foundation, you can watch it at https://bdd-foundation.org/lockdown-webinars-emdr-as-a-treatment-for-bdd

Chapter 13

Using the Voice Dialogue Approach with People Experiencing BDD

———

JOACHIM SCHNACKENBERG AND NICOLE SCHNACKENBERG

Most of us are familiar with conflictual feelings when making decisions. It is also a common human experience to feel surprised by how emotionally charged our reactions are in certain situations. Continuing an argument inside our heads, long after the argument with another person is over, is also perhaps familiar to most of us, as is trying to change a habit while part of us still strongly desires the thing we are trying to stop or give up. In the context of body dysmorphic disorder (BDD), a part of the person may wholeheartedly believe the perceived appearance flaw or defect is real and just as awful as they view it to be, while another part of them wonders if their struggle may be emotional, not physical, in nature (i.e. wondering if they are experiencing BDD). It may also seem as if the 'BDD part' of the person is encouraging them to focus entirely on their making it difficult for them to focus on other things. This appearance-focused part may then be interpreted by the person and others as the enemy. These experiences, and many besides, are relevant to an approach known as Voice Dialogue.

Voice Dialogue hypothesises that we are all made up of numerous inner personalities, parts or selves (Kent, 2019; Stone & Stone, 1998). This is not, as is sometimes depicted in psychological or psychiatric literature, a sign of illness or psychological distress, but rather an intrinsic element of what it is to be a human being. In this chapter we will explore the potential benefits Voice Dialogue may have to offer to those experiencing BDD.

The Origins of Voice Dialogue

The roots of Voice Dialogue are very much situated in the personal experience and lived application in practice of its founders and discoverers, Hal and Sidra Stone (1998, 2007). Hal and Sidra were working as senior psychologists and therapists when their joint exploration of creative imagination and visualisation, which had started in the early 1970s, moved on to a range of new practice-based insights which seemed to be highly relevant to many aspects of human relationships and conflicts. Hal asked Sidra one day to *become* her vulnerability rather than just talking about it. She promptly moved into a posture and position in the room embodying this vulnerability, going on to see and experience the world as a small child. This had previously been a concept Sidra was more theoretically than practically familiar with via her training in psychology. Both Hal and Sidra were surprised to find that Hal ended up relating to what seemed to be a person who had transformed into a young child, taking on their experience, behaviour and language through the body of the grown-up Sidra. Sidra was surprised to find that she had not simply been acting 'as a child' nor was this child simply an inner concept. Rather, this child appeared to be well and living inside of her. This inner child was a stark contrast to her typical persona as a rational, sensible, in-charge, in-control kind of person.

When Sidra and Hal changed roles, with Sidra relating to Hal's inner child (who was similarly real and present), they knew they were on to something. In their ongoing practical exploration, it became clear to them that there were many different selves within them, each with their own personalities and histories. They also discovered some patterns, rules and dynamics at play. After marrying in 1977, their journey of discovery was further enhanced by their joint realisation that they were arriving at the same kinds of conflicts with each other in their marriage as in their respective previous marriages (both had been married once before). At that point, rather than separating, as may have been their natural inclination at the time, their intrigue as to what was happening won them over. They realised that here, too, different selves were at play – this time showing up through their romantic relationship. Their joint exploration led to some exciting insights and new practices, including: the Psychology of Selves (particularly primary and disowned selves); Voice Dialogue facilitation; the Aware Ego Process; and the phenomenon of bonding patterns (Stone & Stone, 2000, 2007). This chapter will focus on the relevance of the Psychology of Selves and Voice Dialogue facilitation to the experience of BDD.

The Psychology of Selves: Primary and Disowned Selves

A core tenet of the Psychology of Selves approach is that human beings tend to endorse (consciously, semi-consciously or unconsciously) some parts as belonging to them (primary selves) while rejecting others (disowned selves). The endorsement of some parts and the rejection of others can lead a person to over-identify with some parts and under-identify with others. This, in turn, can create what Hal and Sidra refer to as blind spots and painful imbalances, which can be experienced emotionally, physically, psychologically and spiritually.

Voice Dialogue facilitation accompanies a person in the process of becoming experientially aware of, and potentially embracing, all the selves within them, including (and perhaps especially) the selves which have been disowned. The result can be a greater conscious embracing of all the selves in a more aware manner, thus creating greater freedom of choice regarding which part to use and how much, rather than being dominated or feeling one's life is run by one part or another. Thus, the process also promotes a person's felt sense of wholeness and a richer, thicker narrative of who they are and can continue to evolve to be.

The endorsement of or identification with certain selves and the rejection of others should not be confused with a liking or not liking of certain selves, though this may also be the case for some people. Rather, people develop primary selves (or parts) which represent the more dominant aspects of their personalities (which they may or may not like) to protect the vulnerability we all have from birth. This is particularly obvious in one's early years when human beings are significantly dependent on their main caregivers, as you will have read about in Chapter 2. Vulnerability in the context of Voice Dialogue not only relates to the potential of being attacked or similar, but also to one's openness to one's own and other people's realities, independently of potentially negative consequences (Pangaia, 2012).

Primary selves tend to be good at working out what a person needs to do to obtain attention, approval and affection and thus protect their vulnerability and keep them safe. This protection is necessary as the feeling of vulnerability can be experienced with both terror and loneliness, making it difficult to endure for any length of time. Naturally, every human being has experiences associated with vulnerability, and primary selves try to keep out feelings and parts which are associated with these experiences. As a result, vulnerable parts of the person, alongside parts deemed to be poor at protecting their vulnerability (often opposite parts to the primary selves) might become disowned and largely unconscious: that is, not lived out or hidden behind the primary selves, as the primary selves will consider them to be too dangerous. For example, a person might experience a (spoken or unspoken) rule in their childhood, something like, 'One must always be nice and not disagree with one's parents, nor show any anger.' This may lead the child to the conclusion that the aspects of themselves which are, for example, conformist and mellow are welcome. On the other hand, the angry and rebellious parts may be pushed down. In this way, the child learns to identify and thus operate with the 'fawning' parts (that is, the parts which are appeasing, pleasing and pacifying towards a perceived threat) and not give much or any space to the 'boundary-asserting' or 'non-conformist' parts.

Thus, people develop primary selves in response to their experiences, and the principal job of these primary selves is to protect their vulnerability. When a person decides, whether consciously or unconsciously, that they like a certain part (such as the part that is always nice to people) or do not like a certain part (such as the part that does not care about what others think) this does not mean that these parts are genuinely better or worse than others. If one engages with each of these different parts experientially – which is what Voice Dialogue facilitates a person to do – it would likely become clear that all parts of the person are ultimately there to help them to become more fully and authentically themselves. The person may then discover that each part is, in its own way, convinced by its particular way of being and has a meaningful, relevant and potentially life-giving function.

Issues particularly arise when people become identified with certain primary selves and when these selves 'run the show' without the person's conscious awareness. Alongside this, much energy may be spent on keeping disowned selves at bay. This can lead to an imbalance and reduce a person's ability to deal with the many challenges posed by life. It also seems to hold true that no parts of the self like to be locked away in solitary confinement (to use an image offered by Hal and Sidra Stone). 'Locked-away' parts may therefore struggle for a place in the person's consciousness in all sorts of ways as a result, for example, through dreams, daydreams and fantasies, and through the kind of people they find themselves attracted to or feel strongly abhorred by.

When space is not provided in a person's consciousness and awareness for their vulnerabilities and disowned selves, the primary selves may become particularly strong. While primary selves are there to protect the person, in such a situation they can end up taking over in a way which does not feel particularly free anymore. In the context of BDD, an appearance-focused primary self may end up running the show in order to protect the person from, for example, disowned shameful and frightened parts, whose presence threatens unbearable feelings of vulnerability (at least from the perspective of the appearance-focused primary self).

Aims and Facilitation of the Voice Dialogue Approach

The aim of Voice Dialogue is for the person to both experience and become more aware of the different and regularly opposite selves within them and their functions. Change (including therapeutic change; that is, distress-alleviating change) may happen in the process, but this is not Voice Dialogue's stated aim. Such change is more likely to come about not by a new cognitive insight (though such insights regularly occur in sessions and can be illuminating) but simply through the process of allowing, experiencing, acknowledging and witnessing the different parts, thereby enabling them to feel validated and heard. Importantly, Voice Dialogue assumes that none of the parts are intending to be harmful to the person. None, therefore, are in themselves a sign of illness either.

At the same time, Voice Dialogue recognises that people can get stuck in the way they relate to and endorse some of the parts of themselves and not others. It also acknowledges the well-intended motivation of each part and the overtly protective function of many parts (particularly primary selves), including the parts which are seemingly critical of the person. For example, in BDD, feelings of shame may have been disowned so significantly, with little or no space given to the associated feelings of vulnerability, that the preoccupation with one's appearance may feel, and indeed be, protective in some way.

When facilitating the process of Voice Dialogue, some basic rules are helpful to understand and apply:

- Having informed the person about the approach, it is generally helpful to begin by verifying with the person that they truly wish, and give their consent, to engage in the process. It is good practice – particularly if the facilitated person is not well known to the facilitator – to first ask the part or self who knows whether it is safe to engage in the process if the session can go ahead (this is usually a highly protective part).

- It is beneficial to be guided by the naturally unfolding process, rather than forcing it into any particular direction: to hold in mind that there is an innate wisdom at hand which guides an organic growth process.

- It is generally true that a primary self will appear first. Even if a person wishes to go straight to a disowned self, it would still be good practice to engage with a primary self first. Primary selves appreciate being heard and acknowledged before other parts are explored, as they have been working so hard to keep the person safe in some way.

- It is helpful to remember that all parts of the person are ultimately aiming for the person to succeed in life, including the disowned parts. While the primary selves may judge some disowned parts to be bad or dangerous, this does not mean they are dangerous or bad in nature.

- The process of Voice Dialogue is ultimately about increasing awareness of the different parts, via a greater experience of the selves, so the person can have more choice, freedom and balance in how they make use of all their selves.

- To facilitate an increased awareness of the various parts, the facilitator holds the centre position from where the exploration begins, and energetically connects with the various parts from there.

- The process benefits from engaging with opposite parts at different stages, e.g. engaging first with a primary self who is trying to control the appearance and then with a naturally occurring opposite disowned part, which might for example be feeling frightened or shameful.

- It is important to separate again from the different parts at the end of the session. This is helped by the facilitator asking the facilitated person at the end of the process to go into a witness position from where they can hear and see the facilitator briefly summarising (not interpreting) what they have seen and heard during the process.

- An important understanding for facilitators to hold in mind and heart throughout the session is that selves – just like people – have their own personalities, histories and ways of looking at the world.

- The facilitation process is naturally helped by the facilitator connecting also with each arising parts' energies in themselves, without imposing their experience of this on to the facilitated person. It is important for facilitators to hold in mind that parts of themselves they have not yet made space for cannot be easily facilitated in another person, e.g. it is difficult to facilitate a shameful part in another person if the facilitator has not made space for and acknowledged the shameful parts within themselves.

As mentioned earlier in the chapter, locked-up selves will attempt to escape from their 'prison' via any means available. Until they are free to exist in a person's life, these parts may even seem to turn a bit nasty in their language and behaviour in a bid to protest their ongoing unjustified imprisonment. For example, a disowned angry self may come out strongly when a person is very stressed or drunk – or in the context of BDD, when the person stands in front of the mirror. Disowned parts can also go a bit 'wild' when they are finally given a bit of freedom, particularly if this freedom has been prohibited for a long period of time. For example, when a person begins to stand up for themselves and state their boundaries – which is also the natural territory of the angry parts – they may, at the beginning and at certain other times, end up doing so in an over-the-top kind of way.

Another insight offered by Voice Dialogue is that people endorse and reject certain parts not only within themselves, but also within others. When a person judges another person, they are typically making this judgment from the position of a primary self. Therefore, the anger a person finds unbearable and judges in others may be an indicator of suppressed and rejected anger within themselves. Equally, the self-confidence a person finds magnetic in others may highlight a past and/or present pushing down of one's belief in oneself (Pangaia, 2012).

A Typical Voice Dialogue Session

In the practice of Voice Dialogue, a facilitator will sit opposite the facilitated person and invite an open, exploratory, gentle and boundaried engagement with some of their parts. As mentioned earlier, it is good practice (especially if the person is not well known to the facilitator) to initially engage with the part who knows whether it is safe to engage in the session. The facilitator might ask the person where and in which position they sense this part in the room. The facilitator then invites the person to move into that position (sitting, standing, lying etc.).

Once the person has taken on the position of the part who knows whether it is safe to engage, the facilitator attempts to strike up an engagement with that part by connecting with those energies in themselves. The Stones refer to this as an energy dance. Typically, the facilitator engages with and/or speaks with each upcoming part directly, for example, speaking to a protective part by asking questions like:

- So are you the part who knows whether it is safe for Peter to engage in this Voice Dialogue process?

- Is this the main thing you do, or do you undertake other tasks?

- How do you accomplish this? For example, what kinds of tools do you use to do this?

- Does Peter know about you and the kind of work you are doing?

- How much of the time are you there? How much of Peter do you fill with your energy?

- What caused you to come into Peter's life? What would happen if you were not in Peter's life?

- Have you got a message for Peter?

- Is it okay for Peter to engage in this Voice Dialogue process? Have you got any particular concerns about it?

- How would I know if you felt that we should stop with the Voice Dialogue session? How will you let me know?

- Finally, what may I call you?

These questions are adapted from Kent & Zimmerman
(2022) and based on the authors' practice.

Once the facilitated person appears to have a richer sense of this protective part and, crucially, the go-ahead from this part for the Voice Dialogue process to continue, the facilitator asks to speak to the person back in the original 'centre' position, ensuring the person has separated from the previous self. From there, a similar process can be engaged with again, focusing on any emerging primary and/or disowned selves. It is important for the facilitator to follow the natural process of the parts arising rather than predetermining the process or having a set plan for the session beforehand. Throughout, the facilitator and the facilitated person ideally remain open to stopping the process or taking a break if they sense it might be getting too much or if the protective part (spoken to at the beginning of the process) somehow intervenes and makes it clear that it no longer feels comfortable or safe to continue.

At the end of the session, the facilitator summarises what they have witnessed from a witness position (sometimes called the witness statement). The facilitator asks the facilitated person to stand next to them, facing out towards the room together, as the facilitator briefly describes what took place during the session from the facilitator's perspective. A Voice Dialogue session should normally not exceed around 90 minutes and can be shorter. Voluntariness of engagement is naturally paramount throughout the process.

During the Voice Dialogue process with people experiencing BDD, people will often refer to a BDD part or similar. However, in reality, the BDD part can be helpfully further differentiated into a myriad of parts. Typically, these might include frightened parts, vulnerable parts, appearance-focused parts, self-critical parts, protective parts and shameful parts. Therefore, it can be helpful when facilitating the Voice Dialogue process with someone experiencing BDD to explore each of these parts in turn, rather than jumping straight to 'BDD' as if it were one singular, separate part. Below are some questions which may be helpful as part of this process (adapted from Kent & Zimmerman, 2022; with the addition of some from our own practice):

- When did you come into Susan's life?

- What was happening in Susan's life at that time which made you feel you needed to come?

- What is your purpose in Susan's life currently?

- How do you do that? What techniques do you use?

- How do you feel about the responsibilities etc. you have in Susan's life?

- What might have happened if you had not come into Susan's life?

- If you were not able to do your job or were not there in Susan's life, what do you feel might happen to her?

- Are there other parts of Susan you are aligned with? How do you connect/work together?

- Are there any parts of Susan you are afraid of and/or wish were not there? Why?

- Are you connected to Susan's preoccupation with aspects of her physical appearance (with her BDD)? If so, how?

- How do you view Susan's BDD [or use whichever term the client uses for their appearance-focused distress]?

- What is the most pressing and important message you want to give Susan today about yourself? And about Susan and her life in general?

A vital element of Voice Dialogue is the facilitator's capacity, openness and willingness to feel different parts and aspects within themselves. If, for example, a quiet, hesitant and frightened child part comes up in a session, the facilitator remains open to both feeling this part within themselves and to expressing empathy for this part in the other person by channelling quiet, hesitant and frightened child energies within and from themselves. At the same time, the facilitator maintains an awareness of the process from the centre position; that is, they refrain from getting lost in the energy of a part within themselves entirely. An easy mistake for facilitators to make can be to slip into a protective or mothering part. However, it is not the aim of Voice Dialogue to therapise or fix the person. 'Facilitate, don't fix' is a central motto of the approach.

Practice Example

The following short practice example is an amalgam of various sessions we have facilitated with people struggling with BDD over the years. It details a facilitation with one of the parts relevant to BDD, which in this case is initially referred to as 'Ugliness'. Details have been changed to respect and protect anonymity.

After seeking permission from 'Farah's' part who knew whether it would be safe to engage in the session, Farah connected with her felt sense of ugliness which she called, and agreed for the facilitator to call, simply 'Ugliness' for ease during the session. Farah sensed Ugliness to be cowering in the corner of the room. Thus, Farah took on a cowering position in the corner of the room and felt into the associated sensations in her body related to Ugliness with the help of the facilitator. She felt Ugliness particularly in her face and chest, in the area of her heart. After a period of both the Voice Dialogue facilitator (VDF) and Farah's Ugliness part sitting in silence together, as Ugliness did not appear to want to speak for a while, the Voice Dialogue moved on to a speaking process:

VDF: Hello. Are you the part of Farah she calls Ugliness?

Ugliness: Yes.

VDF: It is good to meet you. How are you?

Ugliness: I'm scared.

VDF: Yes. It is all very scary.

Ugliness: Yes. Farah doesn't like talking about me. She worries that if she talks about me, you will notice how ugly she is too.

VDF: And how about you? Are you worried about that?

Ugliness: I'm scared but primarily I'm just trying to do my job.

VDF: So, you are scared, but you also have a job to do. What is your job?

Ugliness: I point out to Farah that some of her physical features do not look right or sometimes are even detestable and ugly.

VDF: And how did you realise you needed to do that?

Ugliness: Well, I saw that Farah needed to focus on something she could change to make herself feel safer.

VDF: I see. So, it is important for Farah to feel safer?

Ugliness: Yes. Well, she has been unsafe in the past. She always felt at risk of losing the love of those most important to her if she couldn't be good enough. She is still stuck in those feelings. She believes every person she meets or is connected to will ultimately reject her.

VDF: So, things are still quite difficult for Farah. That must be very frightening for some parts of Farah.

Ugliness: It is. Parts of Farah are terrified. Other parts feel full of shame because they believe Farah is bad in some way.

VDF: I see. And what is your view of the parts of Farah which are terrified and full of shame?

Ugliness: I think that without me those parts would swallow her up.

VDF: So, you stop shame and terror from swallowing Farrah up?

Ugliness: Yes. That is my job: to protect Farah from those parts.

VDF: Wow. It sounds like you are doing an extremely important job by protecting Farah from those feelings of shame and fear. And if for whatever reason you were not there to protect her, what would that be like for Farah?

Ugliness: I dread to think what would happen if Farah didn't have any hope that there might be a way to become good and lovable in the eyes of others.

VDF: Yes. You are doing a truly existentially important job. Has your job always been so important in Farah's life? What made you come into Farah's life in the first place?

Ugliness: Farah was five years old. She was feeling like she wasn't good enough – for her parents, her grandparents, her teachers... She tried so, so hard yet was so often treated like a 'bad girl'. It was so confusing for her. The world seemed like a scary and unpredictable place.

VDF: So, you came along?

Ugliness: I did. I was there in the background at first. Then, later I told Farah she was being treated unkindly and was feeling not good enough, even bad, because her skin was blemished. I told her if she could change the way she looked, she would be treated kindly and people would love her. I told her that if she 'fixed' her skin, she would feel good enough and everything would be okay.

VDF: I see. And how did you know that that was what Farah needed?

Ugliness: Farah needed a project – something to hold on to. She needed something she could take control of and work on, so she didn't disintegrate into hopelessness and shame and despair completely.

VDF: Is that what would have happened if you hadn't come along? That Farah would have disintegrated into despair?

Ugliness: Yes. I think Farah would have thought she was a bad and unlovable person without knowing why and feeling there was nothing she could do about it. So, I told her there was something she *could* do about it. If her skin was nice and smooth, everything would be okay!

VDF: So, you gave Farah hope?

Ugliness: I gave her something to hope for, yes. Without that, I think she would have given up on life. Given up on herself.

VDF: I see. Thank you for explaining that. You indeed have an extremely important role in Farah's life. You have been giving her hope so she believes one day she will feel lovable and good.

Ugliness: Yes. That's what Farah yearns for more than anything else in the world. To feel lovable and good. This whole thing has never been about her skin at all.

VDF: Thank you. You have shared some very important insights with us today. You have also explained how it is very intensive work for you. What would have to happen for you to be able to do a little less? Or to use your energy in a different way?

Ugliness: Well, I wouldn't need to protect Farah from her shame if she came to realise that this feeling was born out of the way she was treated – not because she is 'bad' in some way. She would come to realise she *is* good enough, and always has been.

VDF: Thank you. I appreciate you explaining how important it is for Farah to understand her intrinsic goodness. We are coming to the end of our time together today. Before we finish for now, I am wondering – is there another name you would like to be called or does Ugliness feel right to you?

Ugliness: I have been labelled as 'Farah's felt sense of ugliness' for so long. I would like to be called 'Defender of Worthiness'.

VDF: Thank you Defender of Worthiness. Thank you for working so hard to help Farah not to lose hope. It was very good to connect with you today. And when you are ready, can I speak to Farah in the centre [that is, the original chair position] again?

The facilitation process then goes on to accompany the person in re-centring back in the original chair position and gently separating (not pushing away) from the part they have been exploring. Following this, the facilitator may explore another naturally arising part/self (such as the disowned, shame part) or, if the person feels it is good to finish, the session may end there with the witness statement. In our experience of facilitating the 'Shame' part in people experiencing BDD, Shame often ends up explaining (in some way or another) that they are not there to make the person feel bad. Rather, Shame would appear to be there to alert the person to the ways in which they have been treated unkindly, humiliated, ignored and/or loved conditionally by significant others.

Following the completion of the Voice Dialogue process it would not be unusual for Farah to express a sense of relief for having given space to these parts and an enhanced realisation of their respective good intentions.

We can see from this facilitation process that 'Ugliness' (or, rather, 'Defender of Worthiness') had some valuable information to share with and for Farah, and seemed relieved to be heard and acknowledged. It may be that some change happens simply as a result of the facilitation process. For example, Ugliness may no longer feel quite so pushed aside and, thus, make less virulent attempts to be heard. Other primary selves, such as a self-critical part, may no longer feel such an urge to protect Farah from her feelings of shame and unworthiness as a result. We can also glean from this dialogue that the true intention of Ugliness is to protect Farah and to offer her an avenue of hope and, ultimately, healing. It is also worth noting that the emergence of the 'Defender of Worthiness' (Ugliness) part at the age of about five may indicate an experience or experiences of, for example, bullying, constant questioning of her worth by significant attachment figures, sexualised violence, highly unpredictable and aggressive/withdrawn/emotionally unavailable caregivers or similarly painful experiences. While it may be beneficial for Farah to acknowledge what happened at some point, it may be even more important to explore and experience the unacknowledged feelings/energies any such vulnerable experiences left her with.

Insights like these can feel enlightening, relieving and promising. People often positively comment on Voice Dialogue's non-pathologising and/or non-problematising stance, appreciating its lack of attempt to get rid of any parts or aspects of themselves. As with other approaches, it will ultimately be for Farah to decide if she wishes to implement any changes as a result, i.e. whether she wants to make time to listen, feel into and share with trusted others what Ugliness and/or Shame might have to say; whether she is open to exploring ways of soothing Ugliness's intensity by spending more time with her feelings of shame and her vulnerability and so on. This, in turn, will likely pave the way for other parts of Farah who have had little chance to come through, such as hopeful, boundary-setting and freedom-loving parts.

Concluding Reflections

From a Voice Dialogue perspective, it is not the respective parts, nor indeed whether they are primary or disowned, who are the source of the 'issue'. Instead, it is the imbalanced and non-aware relationship a person has with parts of themselves which can create difficulties in everyday functioning, including in the context of the experience of BDD.

Importantly, although Voice Dialogue may come across as having a strong psychological foundation, Hal and Sidra Stone are clear that it is not a 'therapy'. As such, one does not need to be a formally trained therapist to apply Voice Dialogue facilitation. However, there is a clear recommendation that the process necessitates a degree of training with experienced facilitators and trainers and ongoing personal work (particularly of being facilitated oneself) to be able to offer it in practice. Application in the mental health field is also best carried out by facilitators who have experience and understanding of the presenting mental health struggle of the facilitated person. You can read about this in more detail in the International Voice Dialogue Agreement (IVDA, 2008).

The number of psychiatric and psychotherapeutic professionals applying the Voice Dialogue approach within mainstream mental health services unfortunately appears to be limited at the time of writing, including in the context of the experience of BDD. We hope this chapter has demonstrated the potential benefits of this approach to people experiencing a distressing preoccupation with their appearance, and invites further exploration for some readers.

This chapter has explored just some of the possibilities Voice Dialogue may offer. In the context of BDD, just like with any mental health presentation, a key insight is that the experience is composed of numerous frightened parts of the self which are attempting to protect the person in some way. When heard, understood and validated, these parts can relax and return to their naturally valuable state, thereby themselves becoming a conduit towards healing, wholeness and freedom.

References

IVDA (2008). International Voice Dialogue Agreement. Accessed 08/08/2022 at www.ivda.info

Kent, J. (2019). *Selves in action: How different parts of us inform and influence our daily lives*. John Kent Publications.

Kent, J., & Zimmerman, M. (2022). *Facilitator training. Workshop 1: The basics (including the inner critic)* (Handout). Voice Dialogue UK.

Pangaia, J. O. (2012). *An introduction to voice dialogue: Finding the benefit of people who bug you*. Heart of the Garden Publishing.

Stone, H., & Stone, S. (1998). *Embracing our selves*. New World Library.

Stone, H., & Stone, S. (2000). *Partnering: A new kind of relationship. How to love each other without losing yourselves*. Nataraj Publishing.

Stone, H., & Stone, S. (2007). *The basic elements of voice dialogue, relationship, and the psychology of selves: Their origins and development.* Accessed 19/08/2022 at www.voicedialogue.tv/the-basic-elements-of-voice-dialogue-relationship-and-the-psychology-of-selves-10-part-series-part-1-hals-earliest-influences-and-experiences

Chapter 14

Imagery Rescripting for BDD

———

ROB WILLSON

Mental images are more than pictures in our minds. While mental images often take a visual form, they may include other sensory modalities as well such as the auditory, olfactory or kinaesthetic (Kosslyn, Ganis & Thompson, 2001). The bodily sensations component of mental images can be powerful in body dysmorphic disorder (BDD). For example, a person who has a mental image of their face sagging on one side might have a strong physical sensation accompanying it, making the image seem far more real to them. Moreover, mental imagery has a higher impact on one's emotional state than verbal thoughts, and distressing memories are far more likely to present as images (Hirsch & Holmes, 2007).

Imagery Rescripting (IR) was originally developed for PTSD (post-traumatic stress disorder) (Smucker & Niederee, 1995) and personality disorder (Arntz & Weertman, 1999). It involves modifying distressing mental images or constructing new positive images in ways which help the person feel better. Several years ago, I was encouraged to apply IR through my experience of two workshops: one run by Anne Hackman, Emily Holmes and James Bennett-Levy; and another by Arnoud Arntz. In both cases, I was immensely inspired to hear how accomplished clinicians were being guided by creativity and a determination to help their clients feel better, rooted in a developing science.

This chapter will explore how IR might be applied with individuals experiencing BDD.

Mental Imagery in BDD

In a study conducted by Osman et al. (2004) which compared 18 people diagnosed with BDD and 18 controls, it was found that both individuals with BDD and controls were just as likely to experience spontaneous images of their appearance. However, those with BDD were found to experience appearance-related images which were significantly more negative, more recurrent, and viewed more from an observer perspective (seeing themselves in their mind's eye from another person's viewpoint) than were those of the controls. In the BDD group, the content of the images was frequently related to early aversive memories from childhood or adolescence. The most common memories were of bullying or teasing.

These findings were confirmed by Buhlmann et al. (2007) and Buhlmann (2011), who also found that people with BDD reported a greater number of memories of appearance- and competency-related teasing than did control participants. Neziroglu, Khemlani-Patel, & Yaryura-Tobias (2006), in a sample of 50 individuals with BDD, found that 38 per cent had experienced some form of sexual, physical or emotional abuse. Importantly, Cooper & Osman (2007), in a sample of 18 people diagnosed with BDD, found evidence of increased self-consciousness and decreased self-confidence, alongside negative self-judgments such as being ugly, inferior or worthless.

The prevalence and impact of mental imagery in BDD would seem to suggest that imagery might be a prudent target for treatment in psychological therapy.

Empirical Support for Imagery Rescripting

There is empirical data to support the efficacy of IR in the treatment of a broad range of clinical presentations (Hirsch & Holmes, 2007; Stopa, 2011). Examples of areas in which IR has been applied and demonstrated to have beneficial outcomes include:

- Snake fear (Hunt & Fenton, 2007).

- Obsessive compulsive disorder (OCD) (Veale et al., 2015).

- Survivors of childhood sexual abuse (Smucker et al., 1995).

- Personality disorders (Arntz, 2011).

- Depression (Brewin et al., 2009).

- PTSD (Hackmann, 2011).

- Social phobia (Wild & Clark, 2011).

For a detailed discussion and description of imagery work with a variety of clinical presentations, the reader is encouraged to consult Hackmann, Bennett-Levy and Holmes (2011).

There is also evidence to support the use of IR when working directly with people diagnosed with BDD. For example, Ritter & Stangier (2016) classed four out of six people with a diagnosis of BDD as treatment responders following IR. In our 2016 study (Willson, Veale & Freeston, 2016), we also found that four out of six participants achieved clinically significant change. It should be noted that all the people who were invited to participate in our trial could identify aversive memories connected to their BDD.

In the light of recent moves by many therapists to working online, it is of note that Paulik et al. (2021) found IR by telehealth to be no less effective than face-to-face delivery. They did, however, report that some people found practical limitations, such as a lack of privacy, to be a hindrance in some way. Promisingly, Pennesi and Wade (2018) found that online-adapted IR was effective in improving body image acceptance in a non-clinical sample of young women.

However, in a recent randomised controlled trial, Ghaderi et al. (2022) did not find evidence of a significant positive impact of IR on body-image dissatisfaction. Clearly further trials of IR for BDD and related struggles are needed. Nevertheless, therapists and other professionals supporting people experiencing BDD can be encouraged by the positive outcomes of other studies and anecdotal accounts that IR can be beneficial for those with this diagnosis.

Practical Application of Imagery Rescripting

Across the following pages is a guide to applying IR with a client experiencing BDD, broken down into five main steps. I strongly recommend that your first practice of IR is with a non-clinical volunteer such as a willing colleague, and that you seek clinical supervision from someone practised in the approach.

1. Introduce the Concept of IR and Address Any Doubts and Reservations

First, introduce the concept of IR. A key rationale is that the emotional experiences we have today can sometimes be 'echoes from the past'. IR is an approach which has been designed and tested to help people change the impact of distressing past events. The approach 'does what it says on the tin' and works to rewrite the images associated with memories of aversive events.

Many people with BDD are sensitive to the idea that they might have the 'wool pulled over their eyes', including through fear of the therapist ignoring their distress and struggles. It is, therefore, important to be ready to deal with any reservations your clients may have about changing memories related to their BDD or otherwise. I often explain that the 'knowing' department of their memory bank will still remember what 'really' happened and that we are hoping to improve the images stored so they have a less harmful effect. In this regard, I sometimes share the following personal example of my own rescripted memory with clients:

> The memory I describe is of my younger self, around eight years of age. I was playing with some friends in the playground at school. We were sitting on our favourite spot, on a wall by some steps. For reasons I can't recall, we were pushing and pulling each other, and I accidentally pushed my best friend, Robin, backwards off the (thankfully low) wall. This must have hurt him a fair bit as he sprung back to his feet with utter rage in his young eyes. Realising his fury, I ran for it, but he caught me and pushed me to the ground. He then sat on top of me, grabbed either side of my head with his hands and began repeatedly banging my head on the path beneath. I have a fuzzy idea of someone eventually stopping him, but I can't remember the details. The reason I began to wonder about the relative importance of this memory was that, in my adult life, if ever I banged my head (or someone or something banged it for me) I'd feel intense rage followed by sadness.

In my rescript of this memory, my adult self enters the scene and places a pillow between my head and the paving slabs that made up the path. This instantly reduces the harm inflicted. Next, my adult self pulls Robin off my younger self and calms him. Finally, my adult self helps my younger self up, hugs him and checks he's okay. He then turns to both boys for a bit of a debrief of events so they leave together as friends. I point out to my clients that I retain a clear understanding of what happened in this event, but the images associated with it now are significantly less painful. One of the reasons I think this rescript is of value as an illustration is the pillow: it demonstrates that sometimes the rescript doesn't have to be hugely dramatic, or require profound words to be of impact and value.

Sometimes, I also give a brief explanation of the origin of the IR approach and outline some of the alternative strategies available for dealing with aversive memories. It can also be helpful to use everyday expressions to express the value of working in and with imagery, such as 'a picture paints a thousand words'.

2. Identify a Clinically Relevant Aversive Memory

Assuming your client sees the sense and potential value of using IR, the next step is to agree on a memory to target. The steps below are designed to help a client to identify a memory linked to their BDD. However, some clients will have already discussed a related memory with you or will be quickly able to identify one, in which case the steps below can be edited out as appropriate.

a. Ask your client to provide a recent or representative example of their BDD being activated.

b. Help your client to identify the main emotion they felt such as shame, anxiety, hurt, humiliation etc.

c. Encourage your client to focus on the physical location of the emotion. This might be anywhere in the body. In my experience, however, common areas include the stomach, head, neck, throat, jaw and shoulders.

d. 'Bridge' to a memory – Ask your client: 'What was the first or earliest time you felt this way?' This is very often effective in helping a client to recall a memory related to the emotion identified. If your client has a difficult time identifying an emotion, you can also help them to make a connection ('bridge') from a memory, e.g. 'What's the earliest memory you have of thinking this way?' or 'What's the earliest memory you have of believing...[insert belief]?'

It can be helpful to identify the meaning of the memory with your client and then to return to whether this meaning has changed following the rescript.

3. Rescripting

Having identified a memory related to your client's BDD, check they feel comfortable to proceed to the next step of rescripting (changing and rewriting) the images in their mind from their memory of the experience. In our trial of IR for BDD, the IR had three stages:

a. *Re-live*: Here, ask your client for a description of the memory in the first person, present tense (i.e. their younger self's perspective). It's worth noting that this step alone can sometimes lead to a change in perspective. Re-living is not an essential step, however, and there are times (such as when re-living is likely to be excessively distressing) when it is better not to use it.

b. *Rescript*: Here, typically the adult self enters the 'scene' of the image to intervene or change the ending, offer comfort etc. For example, ask: 'What does your younger self [or 'ten-year-old Amita', say] need to happen here to help them feel better?', or 'Can you make that happen in your mind's eye?' Keep prompting and encouraging your client with such questions to help them to modify the image.

c. *Re-play*: Ask your client to imagine the scene again, but from the younger self's perspective. Ask if there is anything else the person (e.g. the younger self in the memory) needs in order to help them to feel better (and, again, ask your client to imagine this happening). This is often where the most imaginative elements of the rescript emerge.

Some clients find it difficult to imagine their 'older self' entering the scene. It can be helpful to encourage your client to hold their focus on the spirit of the endeavour – to transform the image for the better or create a new one. Anyone kind and helpful could be brought into the image to help. This might include friends, family members, the therapist...and I've certainly known more than one superhero to come to help in an IR.

4. Close

a. Help your client to 'ground' themselves in the current time and place, through grounding practices such as drawing their attention to the sounds they can hear in the room, feeling the floor beneath their feet and the chair under their body, naming five things they can see in the room etc.

b. Check your client's reaction to the rescripting process: What have they made of it? Did anything about it stand out to them?

c. Enquire as to the impact of the IR on the meaning of the memory. Has the strength of belief in the original meaning changed?

d. The choice might then be to stop there and allow time for processing/accommodation or to go on to elicit ideas about how the rescript may help to drive more (life-affirming and supportive) thoughts and/or actions.

5. Follow-Up

During the next session with your client (assuming you have one), check in with their impressions of the IR from the previous session, and any effects they have noticed since. It can be useful to consider how they might now choose to think and act differently in the present to help strengthen or maintain positive changes. In my experience, many clients have returned to the following session with accounts of other memories they have worked on themselves. IR can be used as a brief, standalone intervention, but can also be used over several sessions if your client has multiple aversive memories they wish to target.

Clinical Considerations

When I first started presenting our data and experience of using IR for BDD, I was offered a word or two of caution from some clients and professionals (who were not using the approach). The notion that the therapist might accidentally trigger a dramatic increase in symptoms by working on a person's memories has been a common concern. The fears were largely that post-traumatic stress or similar might be triggered by either 'uncovering' repressed material or by re-traumatising the person. However, it is reassuring and heartening to note that IR has been used for trauma-related experiences for over two decades and has a growing body of empirical research behind it. At the time of writing, I can say that while some clients have not found IR especially helpful, many have, and I've not yet seen anyone become suddenly traumatised as a result.

Naturally, good rapport and a trusting relationship provide a strong foundation for engaging someone in IR. It is important to make sure your client is robust enough to face a difficult memory, and that they can access support if needed. It's also important to be sure to allow enough time in the session to complete the IR. Similarly, leaving enough time to debrief with your client, and supporting them to orientate themselves to the present time and place after the IR, are vital.

It is possible in the process of IR that your client may disclose experiences of childhood abuse or similar traumatic or distressing experiences. Should this arise, it is important to demonstrate sensitivity and professionalism. Help your client to feel safe, respected and as free from shame as possible. A few words of gratitude for the implied respect and trust of the disclosure, as well as showing you really understand their distress as a normal reaction to an 'abnormal' experience, can make a significant difference. All clinicians must of course be mindful of the priority of safeguarding young and/or vulnerable people. You may need to discuss the limits of confidentiality with your client, including that you may need to contact an appropriate organisation or agency if potential risk remains.

IR Example

Below is an amalgam example IR with a client we shall call Dawn who had been experiencing BDD for the past six years and was currently preoccupied with her appearance for more than eight hours a day. Dawn had previously had two trials of CBT, only one of which was partially successful. Dawn's main areas of concern were her skin, eyes and hair. The core distressing emotions driven by BDD were anxiety and shame, especially around others. The impact on functioning of Dawn's BDD was high. For example, preparation of hair, clothing and make-up before leaving the house would take Dawn around five hours. Unfortunately, Dawn had experienced repeated bullying at school, which began in primary school.

IR 1: Kindness, Assertion and a Pot of Paint

Memory: Age nine, Dawn made an extra effort on her hair to make it look pretty, shortly thereafter receiving extreme criticism from a bully in the classroom. Being afraid of this bully themselves, many of her fellow pupils laughed. The class teacher did or said nothing to help.

Meaning attached to memory: *People all agree that I'm ugly and worthless and that I deserve to be put down* (strength of belief: 90 per cent).

Rescript:

- Older self enters the classroom.

- The older self deals with the teacher assertively, admonishing them firmly for not being stronger and more protective.

- Before the bully is aware of what is happening, the older self tips a large pot of paint on the bully's head. The bully is visibly shocked by this. The other pupils laugh and point at the bully.

- The older self takes the younger self aside for a few moments to offer her some comfort and explains the nature of bullying – that it's not her fault but the result of an insecure person enjoying feeling powerful.

Meaning post-IR: Strength of belief in *People all agree that I'm ugly and worthless and that I deserve to be put down* reduced to 40 per cent.

IR 2: Laser-Guns and Play

Memory: Image of the bully walking towards Dawn across the playing field, saying 'You don't want to be near her, she's much too funny looking.'

Meaning attached to memory: *I'm powerless and unwanted because I'm so ugly* (strength of belief: 75 per cent).

Rescript:

- Younger self, not adult self.

- Image of the bully walking towards Dawn across the playing field; her younger self pulls a laser gun out of her pocket and 'zaps' the bully. The bully disintegrates into a cloud of dust.

- The younger self is then invited to play chase with some other children in the playground, who also feel very happy about the bully's fate.

Meaning post-IR: Strength of belief in *I'm powerless and unwanted because I'm so ugly* reduced to 20 per cent. *I really know now that the way I feel about the way I look is more to do with what happened at school than how I look* (strength of belief: 90 per cent).

It's of note here that this is an example of IR seeming to help to support an alternative, psychological explanation of the client's BDD, i.e. helping the client to appreciate that their distress is related to past experiences, not because they are 'ugly' as they previously believed and perceived. It is not unusual for a psychological perspective on an appearance concern to be significantly more credible after an IR demonstrates a difference.

In the following session, the client summed up the effect IR had had on her view of her appearance: *I'm not perfect, but not too bad. You've just got to make the most of what you've got* (strength of belief: 90 per cent). Importantly, Dawn's gains were maintained at follow-up. She went on to make a success of returning to full-time education, with her distress related to her appearance remaining significantly reduced.

Concluding Reflections

IR can be an effective treatment for BDD and has good empirical research support. For some individuals, it can be effective as a brief, standalone intervention (Willson et al., 2016). In their paper on IR for OCD, Maloney et al. (2019) propose that the technique has benefits for individuals who remain symptomatic following a reasonable trial of Exposure Response Prevention (ERP), which is one of the NICE Guideline treatments for BDD. Indeed, my experience has been that the same can hold true for individuals with BDD. Hence, IR may offer an empirically grounded alternative or addition to ERP for BDD alongside the other approaches outlined in this book. The fact that IR can be relatively well-adapted to remote working, including online, further supports its potential.

References

Arntz, A. (2011). Imagery Rescripting for personality disorders. *Cognitive and Behavioral Practice, 18*(4), 466–481.

Arntz, A., & Weertman, A. (1999). Treatment of childhood memories: Theory and practice. *Behaviour Research and Therapy, 37*(8), 715–740.

Brewin, C. R., Wheatley, J., Patel, T., Fearon, P., Hackmann, A., Wells, A., ... & Myers, S. (2009). Imagery Rescripting as a brief stand-alone treatment for depressed patients with intrusive memories. *Behaviour Research and Therapy, 47*(7), 569–576.

Buhlmann, U. (2011). Treatment barriers for individuals with body dysmorphic disorder: An internet survey. *Journal of Nervous and Mental Disease, 199*(4), 268–271.

Buhlmann, U., Cook, L. M., Fama, J. M., & Wilhelm, S. (2007). Perceived teasing experiences in body dysmorphic disorder. *Body Image, 4*(4), 381–385.

Cooper, M., & Osman, S. (2007). Metacognition in body dysmorphic disorder – A preliminary exploration. *Journal of Cognitive Psychotherapy, 21*(2), 148–155.

Ghaderi, A., Welch, E., Zha, C., & Holmes, E. A. (2022). Imagery Rescripting for reducing body image dissatisfaction: A randomized controlled trial. *Cognitive Therapy and Research, 46*, 721–734.

Hackmann, A. (2011). Imagery Rescripting in posttraumatic stress disorder. *Cognitive and Behavioral Practice, 18*(4), 424–432.

Hackmann, A., Bennett-Levy, J., & Holmes, E. A. (eds) (2011). *Oxford guide to imagery in cognitive therapy*. Oxford University Press.

Hirsch, C. R., & Holmes, E. A. (2007). Mental imagery in anxiety disorders. *Psychiatry*, 6(4), 161–165.

Hunt, M., & Fenton, M. (2007). Imagery Rescripting versus in vivo exposure in the treatment of snake fear. *Journal of Behavior Therapy and Experimental Psychiatry*, 38(4), 329–344.

Kosslyn, S. M., Ganis, G., & Thompson, W. L. (2001). Neural foundations of imagery. *Nature Reviews Neuroscience*, 2(9), 635–642.

Maloney, G., Koh, G., Roberts, S., & Pittenger, C. (2019). Imagery Rescripting as an adjunct clinical intervention for obsessive compulsive disorder. *Journal of Anxiety Disorders*, 66, 102110.

Neziroglu, F., Khemlani-Patel, S., & Yaryura-Tobias, J. A. (2006). Rates of abuse in body dysmorphic disorder and obsessive-compulsive disorder. *Body Image*, 3(2), 189–193.

Osman, S., Cooper, M., Hackmann, A., & Veale, D. (2004). Spontaneously occurring images and early memories in people with body dysmorphic disorder. *Memory*, 12(4), 428–436.

Paulik, G., Maloney, G., Arntz, A., Bachrach, N., Koppeschaar, A., & McEvoy, P. (2021). Delivering Imagery Rescripting via telehealth: Clinical concerns, benefits, and recommendations. *Current Psychiatry Reports*, 23(5), 1–10.

Pennesi, J. L., & Wade, T. D. (2018). Imagery Rescripting and cognitive dissonance: A randomized controlled trial of two brief online interventions for women at risk of developing an eating disorder. *International Journal of Eating Disorders*, 51(5), 439–448.

Ritter, V., & Stangier, U. (2016). Seeing in the mind's eye: Imagery Rescripting for patients with body dysmorphic disorder. A single case series. *Journal of Behavior Therapy and Experimental Psychiatry*, 50, 187–195.

Smucker, M. R., & Niederee, J. (1995). Treating incest-related PTSD and pathogenic schemas through imaginal exposure and rescripting. *Cognitive and Behavioral Practice*, 2(1), 63–92.

Smucker, M. R., Dancu, C., Foa, E. B., & Niederee, J. L. (1995). Imagery Rescripting: A new treatment for survivors of childhood sexual abuse suffering from post-traumatic stress. *Journal of Cognitive Psychotherapy*, 9, 3.

Stopa, L. (2011). Imagery Rescripting across disorders: A practical guide. *Cognitive and Behavioral Practice*, 18(4), 421–423.

Veale, D., Page, N., Woodward, E., & Salkovskis, P. (2015). Imagery Rescripting for obsessive compulsive disorder: A single case experimental design in 12 cases. *Journal of Behavior Therapy and Experimental Psychiatry*, 49, 230–236.

Wild, J., & Clark, D. M. (2011). Imagery Rescripting of early traumatic memories in social phobia. *Cognitive and Behavioral Practice*, 18(4), 433–443.

Willson, R., Veale, D., & Freeston, M. (2016). Imagery Rescripting for body dysmorphic disorder: A multiple-baseline single-case experimental design. *Behavior Therapy*, 47(2), 248–261.

Chapter 15

From Fear to Authenticity in BDD

———

TRISTAN KELLER

Considering my own and other people's experience of body dysmorphic disorder (BDD), as well as the available literature on BDD and developmental trauma, I propose the hypothesis in this chapter that BDD is essentially a manifestation of a deep-rooted fear of being oneself. In my estimation, this fear of being oneself is composed of the most fundamental aspects of the human experience, including thoughts, emotions, bodily sensations, perceptions and self-awareness. Therefore, a key aspect of any therapy for BDD would, I propose, helpfully include an exploration of the client's felt sense of authentic, true self, alongside a gentle unearthing of any barriers (past and present) to this true self's full and joyful expression.

Considering the Fear of Rejection and Abandonment

Pervasive feelings of shame are a central characteristic of BDD as you will have read about in other chapters. Included in this experience of shame is a sense that the self is deeply rejectable, and likely to be abandoned by others. Appreciating the deep-rooted fear of rejection and abandonment underlying the experience of BDD – and being aware of how this fuels BDD-related safety behaviours – is essential for therapists working with this client group.

   While the fear of rejection and abandonment is a universal aspect of the human experience to some extent, people with BDD come to a unique way of dealing with this fear. People with BDD tend to believe they themselves are to blame for the neglect, rejection and humiliation they experienced in the past. They internalise feelings of shame, fear and unexpressed emotions such as anger at themselves, which explains the strength of their inner critic and the self-protective parts within them.

People with BDD have typically had early experiences which left them feeling as though it was not permissible, safe even, to be who they are. Somewhere along the line, they will have concluded that they need to change who they are (and what they look like) in order to be loved, and to maintain a relational connection with others (since the alternative of forgoing connection would be too unbearable). In childhood, they may have learned to suppress and inhibit their emotions and to restrict their self-expression, later developing the need to improve or change how they look in a bid to be lovable. The fear of being humiliated and ridiculed may have been stronger than feelings of self-acceptance and authentic expression growing up; therefore, the true self was repressed.

People experiencing BDD ultimately identify their body as the culprit behind dreadful feelings and fears of rejection and abandonment. Their young and vulnerable mind, sometimes as early as in infancy, made a connection at some point in their developmental trajectory: *I need to change how I look in order to avoid rejection and to become lovable.* This conclusion then led to the unfolding of the host of thoughts and behaviours characteristic of the experience of BDD.

Developmental trauma, indeed, appears to be a central aspect of BDD, as you will have read about in Chapter 2. You will also have read about how difficulties with emotional regulation and developmental trauma tend to go hand in hand, including in the context of BDD. People with BDD come to believe their body is the source of their feelings of rejection and shame, correlating their physical appearance (particularly the fixing of their perceived appearance defects or flaws) with feelings of safety and acceptance. Compulsive behaviours are part of the picture, where the safety behaviours (such as mirror checking, mirror avoidance, camouflaging etc.) become the primary means of soothing and of emotional regulation. Therapists working with people experiencing BDD, therefore, would ideally support their client to find alternative, life-affirming ways of soothing the self and regulating painful emotions like shame.

The Foundations of Authenticity and Connection

Regrettably, people experiencing BDD often deem the development of their BDD to be a personal failing. The accompanying logic can be that many people experience rejection, humiliation, teasing or bullying, yet do not go on to develop BDD. The picture, however, is rather more complex than this. There are many factors which contribute to the development of BDD completely outside of the person's control and which help to explain which kind of emotional environment BDD usually thrives in.

There are a myriad of inter-related factors which come into play, creating something of a 'perfect storm' in the development of BDD. People who experience BDD appear to typically possess an innate sensitivity which renders them vulnerable in situations of developmental and complex trauma. Indeed, the majority of people with BDD I've personally encountered have an emotionally sensitive nature. They tend to be thoughtful and compassionate towards others and possess a wide emotional landscape. This emotional sensitivity can be one of their greatest strengths and would ideally be viewed, and explored in therapy, as such.

The downside of this emotional sensitivity is that a turbulent and/or traumatic emotional environment can become rapidly overwhelming. It could be that, due to their innate sensitivity, people with BDD are prone to experiencing emotions more intensely. Thus, the likelihood they will feel overwhelmed or unable to self-regulate difficult emotions may also be greater.

Typically, children learn how to regulate their emotions during infancy, primarily by engaging in co-regulation with their primary caregiver through the process of contingent attunement. This takes place through the numerous emotional interactions between infant and caregiver, and is dependent upon the ability of the caregiver to attune emotionally, moment to moment, to the needs of the child. The process of attunement and containment for the infant happens pre-verbally. Thus, the language young infants speak is an emotional one, orienting themselves towards the tone of voice, eye-gaze and body language of their primary caregiver. The ability of the infant to self-regulate depends first on successful co-regulation: on the primary caregiver's ability to successfully 'read' the infant's emotional states and to attune successfully to their emotional needs. Usually, a primary caregiver and their infant will develop their own 'language', wherein a mother (for example) instinctively knows how to respond to the distress or delight of her infant via various means such as holding the baby, gentle eye-gaze, singing, rocking etc.

There are many factors which can disrupt the process of attunement between a mother or a father and their child. For example, enduring emotional distress or depression of the primary caregiver can interfere with the attunement process, as can familial factors such as transgenerational trauma, poverty, domestic abuse and a lack of community support. If attunement and co-regulation are regularly and consistently impeded, the ability of the child to self-regulate can be impacted also (Maté, 2008).

Without 'good enough' contingent attunement, emotional self-regulation skills can fail to sufficiently develop. Lacking the self-regulatory skills to soothe themselves, these infants can grow into children and later adults without a safe connection to their emotions, and an accompanying sense that any expression of their emotions may be too dangerous or even pointless. As the survival instinct drives the child to maintain connection with their primary caregiver at any price, the child learns to repress their emotions and thereby represses their very sense of self. Over time, the connection to one's authentic sense of self can become minimal or even felt to be lost.

Somewhere along the line, people who experience BDD have learned to suppress their needs, their emotions and, essentially, who they truly are, to maintain a felt sense of connection with others. They may also blame themselves for the lack of genuine connection they experience, adding further evidence to their self-hypothesis that they are 'bad' or 'defective' in some way.

It is possible and plausible that this suppression and internalisation of overwhelming emotions such as fear, shame and anger lie at the root of the development of BDD. Unable to process emotions with an emotionally attuned caregiver, the child's vulnerable mind comes to the conclusion that the child itself is defective or unlovable. This internalised sense of shame, combined with a deep-rooted fear of being oneself, provides a fertile ground, in the fullness of time, for the development of BDD.

The Impact of Developmental Trauma

While the word 'trauma' often evokes mental images of disaster, war or sexual assault, trauma in fact exists on a continuum. Misattunement, emotional neglect, social exclusion, teasing, bullying and humiliation can all have a traumatic impact, depending on the individual and the emotional support systems available to them at the time and thereafter.

Moreover, trauma can also result from 'what didn't happen' (Winograd, 2016). It is possible that certain aspects in childhood which did not occur, and which are crucial for the development of a sense of self, led to the development of BDD for some, if not many, clients. A lack of attunement and adequate emotional nourishment and emotional availability can contribute to an inexplicable sense of loneliness and an inability to process difficult emotions (e.g. shame) effectively.

While it is not a necessary condition for developing BDD, most people with BDD I have met personally have experienced, to some extent, teasing, bullying or humiliation related to their appearance in their childhood or adolescence, or an inflated value placed on appearance in their family system. This lays the groundwork for the pervasive feeling of shame and insecurity that people with BDD so often experience. The message these children and adolescents seem to receive from their surroundings is very clear: *If you look how you look, and if you feel what you feel, you will experience exclusion, humiliation and degradation.* The conclusion can be that if they hide or change how they look, they will finally feel safe and accepted. They will finally feel loved.

The constant fear of humiliation and degradation, paired with an inability to process emotions alone or with an attuned adult, drive the person experiencing BDD to the mirror. The constant mirror checking (or mirror avoidance) and other compulsions are, ultimately, attempts at self-regulation. The price people with BDD pay to feel safe, however, is the connection to their authentic selves.

Moving towards Authenticity

If the fear of being oneself is at the root of the development of BDD, how can clients with BDD be supported to reconnect to their authentic sense of self? If people with BDD experience disconnection from their somatic sensations and emotions, how can they be helped to reconnect with themselves and with the world?

Authenticity is a highly individual process. What feels authentic to one person may feel completely inauthentic to another. Therefore, the process of moving towards authenticity is not one that can be pursued only by cognitive understanding or via the application of certain processes or rules, but rather must include deliberate practice and experience. This involves both trauma-informed and embodied approaches, such as those explored in this book. Supporting clients to develop their awareness of their feelings, thoughts, behaviours and sensations is crucial in the process of greater authenticity and healing. This involves an exploration of emotional regulation in the context of the sensory and nervous systems (see Chapters 5 and 8) and applying genuine self-compassion to one's physical and emotional experience, both current and present (see Chapters 10 and 11). It is crucial, of course, to support clients to develop an attitude of non-judgmental self-awareness towards their felt sense of self.

Clients experiencing BDD can benefit from being supported to acknowledge and witness their emotions and compulsions. Given that the suppression of their emotions and their authentic selves perhaps led to the development of BDD in the first place, suppression may be the person's primary tool when the thoughts and compulsions associated with BDD become overwhelming. Paradoxically, people experiencing BDD also often get told, including by well-meaning mental health professionals, that their feelings and thoughts are 'irrational'; that they should substitute their thoughts for more 'positive' or 'rational' ones. This can further amplify the inner struggle people with BDD experience and feed into their notion that they are defective, and that their emotions are not worth considering and acknowledging.

It is helpful for therapists to remember that while on the surface it appears that people with BDD are afraid of how they look, what they are actually terrified of is the emotions they experience. The overwhelming shame and the fear of rejection they attach to their bodies literally terrorise people with BDD – not the physical-appearance defects or flaws they perceive.

Hence, I firmly believe that the experiencing, acknowledging and releasing of emotions are essential to the healing process in BDD. The suppression of emotions, in fact, is one of the very mechanisms which keeps BDD 'alive'. By developing an attitude of non-judgmental self-awareness, guided by compassion and a genuine willingness to understand one's emotions and experiences, the person can gradually resolve the inner conflict and rediscover their authentic self and rich emotional life.

There are many ways to deliberately practice non-judgmental self-awareness, some of which are offered in other chapters in this book. Many ancient breath-led practices, ranging from yoga to Qi Gong and Tai Chi, require and cultivate an attitude of non-judgmental self-awareness, both on a cognitive and somatic level. Moreover, many sports and art forms, ranging from basketball and tennis, to singing and dancing, to painting and sculpture, require self-awareness as they demand a certain level of skill, technique and control over one's body. When undertaken mindfully, the benefits of such sports and artistic pursuits can become intensified.

Self-awareness encompasses awareness of one's emotions. When sensations and emotions in the body are witnessed and acknowledged within the therapeutic space, they can feel less overwhelming, less frightening and more possible to process and assimilate.

Mindful Self-Compassion

For true healing from BDD to take place, it is necessary for clients not only to become aware of their emotions and learn how to 'tolerate' them, but also to welcome these emotions: to meet them with genuine compassion and understanding. This involves affording clients with the opportunity to tune into their bodily sensations and cognitions; and to attend compassionately to their feelings and needs in the way they would attend to the feelings and needs of a loved one. In my estimation, genuine authenticity and self-hatred are opposed to each other; therefore, the mindful practice of compassionate self-awareness is essential for the cultivation of an authentic self.

Kristin Neff, a renowned researcher in the field of self-compassion, differentiates between the Yin and Yang of self-compassion (Neff, 2019). The Yin aspect of self-compassion can be understood as nurturing, benevolent and understanding, whereas the Yang aspect is supportive, challenging and directed towards the meeting of one's needs. There is no rule of thumb for which kind of self-compassion is most suitable for the experience of BDD, though I suspect people with BDD tend to lack both. The inner critic of the person experiencing BDD tends to be extremely harsh and condemning, pushing them to their psychological limits. Alongside this, people with BDD often lack the ability to set healthy boundaries and to assert their needs.

The struggle to assert their needs can pose a variety of difficulties at work and in relationships for people experiencing BDD. Lacking the defensive and protective benefits of healthy anger, people with BDD are very likely to tolerate unacceptable behaviour and to internalise any accompanying feelings of shame and degradation. Moreover, they may struggle to face day-to-day life challenges, particularly those which require a certain degree of assertiveness. In my estimation, the Yang component of self-compassion is often neglected in therapeutic approaches for BDD. A beneficial element of the therapeutic process for

BDD, therefore, would be to support the client to reconnect with the protective capabilities one's emotions have to offer, and to support them both to recognise and to state their needs and boundaries to others.

Concluding Reflections

Lacking the emotional safety to be themselves, people experiencing BDD repress their authentic self for the sake of maintaining relational connections with others.

If disconnection from the true self and emotional dysregulation indeed lie at the heart of the development of BDD, reconnection with the self and developing one's capacity for emotional regulation are key factors in the healing process. This will not only improve the person's relationship with themselves, but also facilitate, enrich and enliven their relationship with others. Part of the therapist's role, therefore, is to support the client to rediscover who they truly are and to feel safe enough to share their vulnerability, thus facilitating genuine relational connections to emerge and be maintained.

It is also helpful for therapists to remind clients experiencing BDD of the inherent value in their emotions, including the painful, unwanted and difficult emotions. Of course, emotions represent the deepest yearnings of the human heart, such as the need for love, connection and authenticity. To discredit one's inner emotional landscape is to discredit one's humanity, and to cut oneself off from one's authenticity and that of others.

Self-awareness is essential for healing, particularly given that many of the processes which fuel the compulsions and safety behaviours asso-ciated with BDD are unconscious and may stem from early, unprocessed emotions. The self-awareness I am speaking of is one of compassionate inquiry. This is a somatic process, wherein one reconnects with the felt sense of the body, initially beyond the realm of words and explanations. This connection with the felt sense of the body – with one's interoception – is essential within the healing process as you read about in Chapter 5. If somatic self-awareness is paired with genuine self-compassion, true healing becomes possible. Only when all the parts of oneself, including and especially those which have been neglected and suppressed, are listened to and nurtured can the person find a degree of inner peace and wholeness. If this genuine compassion reaches the inner depths, the compulsive thoughts and safety behaviours typical of BDD will slowly diminish by themselves as their *raison d'être* has become obsolete.

Many therapeutic approaches pathologise BDD and focus primarily if not solely on the overt symptoms. I am advocating here that it is important for therapists of any modality working with clients experiencing BDD to step outside of the left hemisphere world of compulsions and cognitions and into an exploration of past experiences of relational trauma alongside: what the person values and cherishes in life; what provides them with a sense of connection and aliveness; what supports them to feel, trust and express their emotions; and, most essentially, who it is they truly are.

Successful recovery from BDD focuses not only, therefore, on what one could helpfully move away from, but also on what one can move towards. After all, life is not about 'not having BDD'. Life is about living, about being one's true, authentic self.

References

Maté, G. (2008). *When the body says no: The hidden cost of stress*. Wiley.

Neff, K. (2019). *The Yin and Yang of self-compassion: Cultivating kindness and strength in the face of difficulty*. Sounds True.

Winograd, A. M. (2016). *Face to face with body dysmorphic disorder: Psychotherapy and clinical insights*. Routledge.

In Closing

NICOLE SCHNACKENBERG, WITH JAMES DOWNS

It feels fitting to close this book with some stirring words about embodiment and body dysmorphic disorder (BDD) from James Downs, mental health campaigner and an expert-by-lived-experience.

We are not just how we think, and our experience – even of mental health problems – is not 'all in our heads'. The mental strife we might go through, including unhelpful ways of thinking we might find ourselves fighting with, are just a part of the picture.

For me, the recognition of the body is something I have often missed when seeking help for struggles with my mental health such as body dysmorphia and eating difficulties. Approaches to helping me overcome my dis-ease or distress have focused heavily on engaging me as a mind – accessed through sitting down and talking and making sense through words. But my ways of being have always been more than just language and words – which is what thoughts are, after all.

My ways of being – however difficult or unhelpful some of them have been – have been more than ways of thinking, but ways of feeling, sensing, experiencing, presenting, changing, moving, and embodying, too. Likewise, there are many ways of knowing and learning – not all of which involve words. Over time I have learnt that each facet of my experience is part of a mosaic-like and ever-shifting bigger picture that makes up the whole of me, and each part deserves attention for what it can reveal and help me to understand.

Embodiment refers to the lived experience of being a body engaged with the world (Piran & Teall, 2012), rather than as a mind, a willpower, an appetite, an image, or a set of thought processes situated in isolation from one another. Embodiment theory reminds us that all human experiences are bodily experiences (Hanna, 2004), and this is never a fixed thing, as much as we might like it to be. Part of what it is to be a body is that it is always moving, always changing, always exchanging – be that on a microscopic cellular level or a grand, visible scale; on the level of the unseen dynamics between us as individuals, or through the cultural or political movements that change the shape of our social world.

Accepting this reality requires us to abandon a degree of self-control and the idea that we as individuals have ultimate power over our actions and path through life.

In my own recovery, surrendering to the idea that there is so much I cannot change has alleviated me of battles that simply aren't worth fighting, and has meant I can find a bit more peace in the everyday. But this has left me wondering whether we really do journey through life at all or whether, instead, the world actually journeys through us, via the gateway of our senses and the vehicle of our bodies.

A consideration of the innate intelligence, wisdom and healing capacity of the 'vehicle of our bodies' has been a central aspect of the chapters contained within these pages. However, much remains unsaid and unwritten. This book has offered just a few of the many possibilities of working with people experiencing BDD and associated struggles through trauma-informed and embodied approaches. I have heard many people in BDD support groups and workshops talk about other modalities they have found helpful which are unfortunately not represented in this book, such as equine therapy, music therapy, sensorimotor psychotherapy, trauma-informed massage, sculpture, creative writing and many others besides. Support groups themselves are very often mentioned by those experiencing BDD as being of significant value in the healing journey. I hope it shall be possible, in the fullness of time, to bring together a second volume to give voice to some of these experiences: of people with lived experience and those supporting them alike.

It is my fervent wish that this book has offered a ray of hope amidst the hopelessness, shame and fear so characteristic of BDD. Hope that there are always options, and a multiplicity of ways of understanding, addressing and soothing the perplexing and seemingly unbearable thoughts, sensations, emotions, memories and experiences related to BDD. And hope also that understanding of, and compassion for, the experience of BDD are steadily increasing, not only through empirical research but also through experts-by-lived-experience and those supporting them informally coming forward with their stories and reflections on what has both hurt and helped them the most.

My sincere and heartfelt thanks go to all the contributing authors of this book, and to the many others who have supported the process, including participants of various BDD support groups who kindly offered their feedback and reflections on some of the content. Your perspective, perceptions, insights and care have been invaluable.

References

Hanna, T. (2004). *Somatics: Reawakening the mind's control of movement, flexibility, and health.* De Capo Press.

Piran, N., & Teall, T. (2012). The developmental theory of embodiment. In G. McVey, H. B. Ferguson, M. Levine & N. Piran (eds), *Improving the prevention of eating disorders: Collaborative research, advocacy, and policy change* (pp. 169–198). Wilfred Laurier Press.

Resources and Further Reading

Resources

- A wealth of information and resources can be found on the BDD Foundation website at www.bddfoundation.org and on the OCD Action website at www.ocdaction.org.uk
- The BDD Foundation now also offer an email helpline: support@bddfoundation.org. More information can be accessed at https://bddfoundation.org/support/online-support/email-helpline
- A card for taking along to GPs and other professionals explaining what BDD is can be downloaded at https://bddfoundation.org/wp-content/uploads/FINAL-GP-CARD.pdf
- A leaflet offering guidance for schools and educational settings supporting young people with BDD can be downloaded at https://bddfoundation.org/wp-content/uploads/BDD-Leaflet-for-Education-Professionals.pdf
- An essay summarising a small-scale, unpublished study (by Richard Cox, 2018) exploring the benefits of meditation for people experiencing BDD can be accessed at www.deepstateconsciousness.com/writing (download the Finding Your Original Face file)
- *EMDR Client Handout*. www.getselfhelp.co.uk
- Find a therapist: https://emdrassociation.org.uk/find-a-therapist
  https://emdrfocus.com/emdr-support/associate-therapists
  www.stillthehunger.co.uk
- EMDR Academy for accredited training: www.emdracademy.co.uk

Suggested Further Reading

Dana, D. (2018). *The Polyvagal Theory in therapy: Engaging the rhythm of regulation* (Norton series on interpersonal neurobiology). WW Norton & Company.

Downs, J., Hopfenbeck, M., Lewis, H., Parker, I., & Schnackenberg, N. (2021). *Practical handbook of eating difficulties: A comprehensive guide from personal and professional perspectives*. Pavilion Publishing.

Fisher, J. (2017). *Healing the fragmented selves of trauma survivors: Overcoming internal self-alienation*. Routledge.

Gilbert, P. (2009). *The Compassionate Mind*. Constable and Robinson Ltd.

Härle, D. (2017). *Trauma-sensitive yoga*. Singing Dragon.

Omer, H. (2020). *Courageous parents: Opposing bad influences, impulses and trends*. MSI Press.

Omer, H. (2021). *Non-violent resistance: A new approach to violent and self-destructive children*. Cambridge University Press.

Omer, H., & Dolberger, D. (2015). Helping parents cope with suicide threats: An approach based on non-violent resistance. *Family Process, 54*(3), 559–575.

Omer, H., Steinmetz, S., Carthy, T., & Schilippe, A. V. (2013). The anchoring function: Parental authority and the parent-child bond. *Family Process, 52*(2), 193–206.

Ona, P. E. Z. (2021). *Living beyond OCD using Acceptance and Commitment Therapy: A workbook for adults*. Routledge.

Rothschild, B. (2000). *The body remembers: The psychophysiology of trauma and trauma treatment*. WW Norton & Company.

Schnackenberg, N., & Petro, S. (2016). *Reflections on body dysmorphic disorder: Stories of courage, determination and hope*. The BDD Foundation.

Schnackenberg, N., Jassi, A., & Monzani, B. (2020). *The parents' guide to body dysmorphic disorder: How to support your child, teen or young adult*. Jessica Kingsley Publishers.

Shapiro, F. (2017). *Eye movement desensitization and reprocessing (EMDR) therapy: Basic principles, protocols, and procedures*. Guilford Publications.

Stone, H., & Stone, S. (1989). *Embracing our selves: The voice dialogue manual*. New World Library.

Van der Kolk, B. (2014). *The body keeps the score: Brain, mind, and body in the healing of trauma*. New York.

Veale, D., Willson, R., & Clarke, A. (2009). *Overcoming body image problems including body dysmorphic disorder*. Robinson Press.

Winograd, A. M. (2016). *Face to face with body dysmorphic disorder: Psychotherapy and clinical insights*. Routledge.

Crisis Helplines

National Suicide Prevention Lifeline (USA): Provides 24/7, free and confidential support for people in distress and prevention and crisis resources.
1-800-273-8255

Papyrus: The UK's leading charity for the prevention of youth suicide.
Hopeline (by Papyrus): A confidential support and advice service for:
- Children and young people under the age of 35 who are experiencing thoughts of suicide.
- Anyone concerned that a young person could be thinking about suicide.

www.papyrus-uk.org
0800 068 41 41
0778 620 9697
pat@papyrus-uk.org

Samaritans: Confidential 24/7 crisis line.
116 123 (no area code necessary)
www.samaritans.org
jo@samaritans.org

SANEline: For people experiencing mental health difficulties or those supporting them.
www.sane.org.uk
0300 304 7000

About the Authors

Jo Dance

Jo trained as a contemporary and ballet dancer and performed and taught dance extensively during her 20s. When she needed something gentler on her body, she studied viniyoga, which she taught for 11 years. Meanwhile, her own health challenges led her to research and explore trauma, natural health and many other holistic modalities, and her four step-children prompted her to delve into peaceful and attachment parenting approaches which she became very passionate about. She has written a book on real food and nutrition, and over the last few years has been campaigning for health freedom and designing ethical clothes that promote love and human connection. She lives in Brighton with her teenage son, close to the sea which they love, and is just starting out as a health coach. You can find her at www.love-tees.me and www.joyfoodrevolution.com

James Downs

James is a mental health campaigner, peer researcher and expert-by-experience in eating disorders. He holds various roles at the Royal College of Psychiatrists, NHS England and a number of universities and charities, all of which focus on developing collaboration across a range of professional and personal perspectives. James is also an Associate Lecturer with the Open University, a Trainee Counselling Psychologist, represents various UK mental health charities, and is a yoga and barre teacher. He has written extensively about his own experiences with the hope that those who read his work find comfort, affirmation and hope.

Rosa Hernando Hontoria

Rosa is an Accredited Cognitive Behavioural Therapy (CBT) Therapist, Compassion Focused Therapist and Mindfulness Trainer. She has worked as a CBT therapist for over 20 years in London and is additionally a Compassion Focused Therapist. Early in her career, Rosa specialised in OCD and BDD and helped in the development of a Highly Specialist Unit for these conditions which receives national referrals from all over the UK.

Rosa has a special interest and extensive training in Third Wave CBT approaches. These include Acceptance and Commitment Therapy and Compassion Focused Therapy, which she is passionate about. She is a trained Mindfulness and Mindful Self-Compassion teacher and believes in integrating body practices in her therapy work with clients. She also specialises in self-esteem difficulties and work with people who have a strong 'self-critic'.

Beverley Hutton

Beverley Hutton is the Clinical Director and Founder of mental health charity Still the Hunger. She is a Psychodynamic Psychotherapist and EMDR Europe Accredited Practitioner, with several years' experience in senior NHS healthcare management. Beverley has a particular interest and experience working with trauma and BDD, dissociative disorders (including dissociative identity disorder) and chronic pain management, and she leads a monthly BDD support group for the BDD Foundation. She previously ran a Therapeutic Community programme for seven years before moving into more individual work with EMDR, which has seen more complex clients being able to make dramatic progress over a much shorter period of time.

She is the author of *Still the Hunger* and *The MORE Course* (both independently published, 2020), which she wrote as a self-help guide for those wanting to understand complex mental health issues from an integrated clinical and spiritual perspective.

Tristan Keller

Tristan Keller is an Integrated Psychological Coach in-training with personal lived experience of body dysmorphic disorder. While having a keen interest in the workings of both body and mind, his original background is in philosophy, politics and economics.

Tristan is currently employed as a social care worker. Curious about the world and the human mind, his interests include Eastern philosophy and neuroscience, as well as trauma-informed therapeutic approaches including Somatic Experiencing and Compassionate Inquiry.

Jill Lubienski

Jill is a Systemic Psychotherapist and Social Worker living and working in Cardiff, Wales. She is an Associate and Accredited NVR Practitioner with Partnership Projects UK, the leading UK provider of Non-Violent Resistance parent therapy, professional training and supervision. Jill also works part time for the NHS as a Family Therapist supporting young people experiencing an eating disorder and their families, in the transition from CAMHS to Adult Mental Health Services. She runs her own independent therapy practice in Cardiff and is mother to two young men.

Jill has an interest in embodiment and trauma and, after many years practising yoga, she recently qualified as a yoga teacher. Jill is also a keen student of Biodanza, a music and movement approach to wellbeing, and of Transcendental Meditation and Ayurvedic integrated health approaches. Jill is delighted to be contributing her particular knowledge, skills and interests to this book.

Dr Alex Mummery

Dr Alex Mummery is an Educational Psychologist working for Haringey Council and an expert-by-lived-experience of BDD. He originally studied Fine Art at the Cambridge School of Art from 2005 to 2007, after which he worked as a Special Needs Teaching Assistant at a North London school for eight years. This experience led him to take a master's course in Educational Psychology at Bristol University, after which he began his doctoral studies at the University College London Institute of Education. In his spare time, he likes to indulge his passion for all things musical and plays the guitar and sings in a number of bands around London.

Joachim Schnackenberg, PhD

Dr Joachim Schnackenberg has been working as a mental health professional in various acute, community and long-term mental health settings since the year 2000, first qualifying as a mental health nurse and later as a social worker. He currently holds the position of Director of Hearing Voices and Recovery in a mental health organisation in Northern Germany.

Joachim also works internationally with the efc Institute (www.efc-institut.de) as a trainer, supervisor, consultant, author and researcher in Experience Focused Counselling with people who hear voices. He is a trained Voice Dialogue facilitator and has experience of applying Voice Dialogue techniques with people with various diagnoses, including people with a diagnosis of BDD.

Dr Nicole Schnackenberg

Dr Nicole Schnackenberg is a child, community and educational psychologist and yoga therapist. She is a trustee of the BDD Foundation and Give Back Yoga UK, and a director of the Yoga in Healthcare Alliance. Nicole is also the founding director of Labyrinth House, a family wellbeing hub in Essex (www.labyrinthhouse.org.uk).

Nicole has authored various books on appearance-focused distress including: *False Bodies, True Selves: Moving Beyond Appearance-Focused Identity Struggles and Returning to the True Self* (Karnac, Routledge, 2016) and *Bodies Arising: Fall in Love with Your Body and Remember your Divine Essence* (John Hunt, 2019). She also co-authored *The Parent's Guide to Body Dysmorphic Disorder* (Jessica Kingsley, 2020), and co-edited *Reflections on Body Dysmorphic Disorder: Stories of Courage, Determination and Hope* (the BDD Foundation, 2016) and *The Practical Handbook of Eating Difficulties* (Pavillion Press, 2021).

Dr Sarah Sivers

Sarah is a child, community and educational psychologist with a commitment to supporting children, young people and those who care for them. She has a particular interest in understanding the lived experience of children and young people and using their views to guide her work. Sarah is passionate about working innovatively and flexibly to find new ways of reaching out to and collaborating with others using psychology. The values that guide her in her work and life are connection, curiosity and authenticity.

She is the co-creator of EP Reach-Out, a webinar series focused on supporting the emotional wellbeing of children, young people, families and educational settings, and the co-author of two chapters in *Children in Lockdown* (Karnac, 2021).

Sarah is a passionate amateur in her journey to develop a deeper knowledge of Acceptance and Commitment Therapy (ACT) and discover how both she and others can lead a more values-guided life. She has been a visiting psychologist and co-facilitator of online BDD support groups where she has trialled and received feedback on some of her ACT practices and exercises for BDD.

Dr Natalie Stechler

Dr Natalie Stechler is a counselling psychologist working at the Nightingale Hospital inpatient Eating Disorder Unit. She also runs a private practice treating a wide array of clients and their needs, and has a breadth of clinical experience from working with body image issues, eating disorders and body dysmorphic disorder, to depression, anxiety, low self-esteem and relationship difficulties. Natalie offers evidence-based therapies including Cognitive Behavioural Therapy, Compassion Focused Therapy, Enhanced Cognitive Therapy and the Maudsley Method of Anorexia Nervosa Treatment for Adults. Her research centres around body dysmorphia and she has recently published a journal article on the relational and interpersonal perspective, including struggles around physically intimate relationships: 'If only he were blind: Shame, trauma, and dissociation among women with body dysmorphic disorder in physically intimate relationships' (*International Journal of Qualitative Studies on Health and Well-Being*, 17(1), doi: 2015871).

Anna Warhurst
Anna is a mental health advocate and expert-by-experience of BDD. She is a Service Designer and Fellow for the Mental Health Collective, an organisation dedicated to finding practical solutions to address the social and collective dimensions of mental health; she has developed and led a number of innovative services and initiatives that aim to increase wellbeing for different disadvantaged groups using co-production methods. Anna is also a meditation teacher, and currently training to become a yoga therapist with the Minded Institute. She is particularly interested in sharing the benefits of yoga and meditation more widely to help people overcome a range of mental health conditions and aid in personal transformation.

Dr Rob Willson
Dr Rob Willson is a cognitive behaviour therapist based in North London, with a special interest in BDD. He is currently the Chair of the Body Dysmorphic Disorder Foundation (bddfoundation.org), the world's first charity exclusively devoted to the condition. Prior to building his own practice, Rob spent 12 years working at the Priory Hospital North London where he was a therapist and therapy services manager. He also trained and supervised numerous CBT therapists over a seven-year period working at Goldsmiths College, University of London. He is regularly invited, around the UK, to train therapists and psychologists in Cognitive Behaviour Therapy for BDD. Rob has co-authored several books, including *Cognitive Behavioural Therapy for Dummies* (John Wiley & Sons, 2019), *Overcoming*

Obsessive Compulsive Disorder (Robinson, 2021) and *Overcoming Body Image Problems Including Body Dysmorphic Disorder* (Hachette, 2012).

Arie Winograd

Arie Winograd, MA, LMFT, has dedicated the vast majority of his career as a psychotherapist to the treatment of body dysmorphic disorder. The Founder and Director of the Los Angeles BDD & Body Image Clinic, he is also the author of *Face to Face with Body Dysmorphic Disorder: Psychotherapy and Clinical Insights* (Routledge, 2016). He regularly lectures and consults on the subject of appearance-focused distress.

Appendix A

Acceptance and Commitment Therapy values cards – drawing upon some ideas from The Happiness Trap values cards (Harris, 2019; see Chapter 10 references).

Honesty To be honest, truthful and sincere with myself and others	**Acceptance** To be open to and allowing of things I don't want or dislike in myself, others and the world around me
Friendliness To be warm, friendly, open, accepting, agreeable and helpful towards others	**Trust** To be trustworthy, loyal, faithful, sincere and reliable; also, to be trusting of others
Integrity To live life with honesty and be guided by my principles and values	**Curiosity** To be curious, open-minded and interested; to be eager to explore, discover and learn new things
Collaborative To engage in shared experiences and projects; to collaborate with others	**Compassion** To act kindly toward myself, others and the world around me; to show empathy
Respectful To treat myself and others with genuine care and consideration; to respect and embrace diversity	**Mindful** To be mindful, open to, engaged in and curious about my here-and-now experiences
Contribution To offer something of myself, give, help, assist, share or be generous	**Organised** To plan, be prepared and think things through carefully; to keep things in order for myself and others

Creativity To be creative and innovative at work and play; to enjoy and promote the creativity of others	**Gratitude** To see joy and wonder in all I see, meet and experience; to show gratitude towards others and myself
Authenticity To be authentic, genuine and real in my approach to life and interactions with others	**Assertiveness** To stand up for my own and other's rights, in a respectful and ethical way
Nurture To care for and hold in mind those around me; to protect and keep others safe	**Optimism** To be hopeful and optimistic about the future and make positive plans
Courage To be courageous or brave; to persist in the face of fear, uncertainty and threatening circumstances	**Forgiveness** To be forgiving toward myself and others; to let go of blame and resentment
Playfulness To be playful, creative and light hearted in my approach to life; to have fun and see the joy in playful moments	**Self-Care** To care for and be kind to myself; to allow myself time to rest and recharge
Flexibility To adjust and adapt readily to difficult or changing circumstances	**Adventurous** To be adventurous; to actively explore new and challenging experiences
Persistence To continue resolutely with tasks or challenges, despite problems, fears and difficulties	**Connection** To engage fully in whatever I am doing; to give the activity, or the person I'm with, my full attention
Responsibility To act responsibly and be accountable for what I do; to take responsibility and think of others	**Supportiveness** To be supportive, helpful and available to myself and others; to encourage and listen
Independence To have the confidence to make my own decisions and follow through on my own plans and ideas	**Your own idea**
Your own idea	**Your own idea**

Appendix B

Butterfly Tapping

With your arms crossed across your chest with your left hand on the right shoulder and right hand on left shoulder, tap your shoulders alternately with your eyes closed. You may notice that your eyes move side to side behind your eyelids as they follow the sound of the tapping and the sensation on your shoulders. Very slow butterfly tapping is used for the Safe Place exercise (see the following page) and for installing the Resource Team. For processing work, the tapping is done at a much faster rate. Butterfly tapping works well for online Eye Movement Desensitisation and Reprocessing (EMDR) sessions.

TouchPoints

These are very clever little devices that can be worn on each wrist during the day or at night to help reduce anxiety, panic attacks and sleep difficulties by calming down the central nervous system. They use BLS with alternating bleeps, vibration and a coloured light to indicate the relevant speed. Most of my clients purchase these devices to use between sessions to manage symptoms on the slow blue setting, and they work for online EMDR sessions on the fast setting. They are not meant to be used for processing without an experienced EMDR therapist alongside. More details about these devices and how to purchase them can be found at www.touchpointeurope.com

Here is a comment made recently by one of my BDD clients who has been using TouchPoints to help with compulsive skin picking between sessions:

> I have struggled with compulsive skin picking for over 25 years; beginning at the age of seven or eight with my arms and legs, then onto my face in adolescence and pretty much every inch of my body by my mid-20s.

I would spend hours every day trapped in a picking state, and when I wasn't, the urge was almost uncontrollable. I started wearing the Touch-Points on my wrists about five months ago and I haven't engaged in a single, prolonged episode of skin picking since. Overall, I would say my picking has reduced by about 90 per cent, which is unbelievable really! I no longer feel like a slave to the tweezers.

Grounding Exercises
These grounding exercises can be tried on your own at home.

The Safe Place
This may be somewhere you have been to before, such as a holiday destination, or it can be entirely imaginary. This place should not have any association to any negative experiences. It is therefore not advisable to use your home, childhood home or bed.

- Bring this place to mind. When you can connect with it, start applying very slow butterfly tapping as described above.

- Notice what you can see in your Safe Place. Notice the colours, the scenery etc. Look around you and take in everything you can see. Continue tapping slowly as you notice what you can see.

- Next, notice what you can hear in your Safe Place. Can you hear waves, trickling water, birdsong, wind rustling leaves? Continue to tap very slowly as you notice what you can hear.

- Now notice what you can feel on your skin. Is it warm or cold? Is there a breeze? Continue with slow tapping.

- Now notice whether there is a fragrance. Can you smell the fragrance of flowers, trees, grass, the sea? Continue with tapping slowly.

- Notice what it feels like to be in your Safe Place. How does it make you feel, and is there a word to describe this place or the feeling? As you tap slowly, repeat the word in your mind and register the feeling in your mind. The word will help you to connect with the feeling when you want to try this exercise again.

Resource Team

If you have experience already of some Compassion Focused Therapy (please also see Chapter 11), you may like to try using this exercise to help you with developing a more compassionate approach towards yourself.

For EMDR we will use three Compassionate/Nurturing Figures, three Protector Figures and one for Wisdom. Some examples may be:

Nurturing/ Compassionate Figure	Protector Figure	Wisdom Figure
Ideal mother	Superhero, Superman etc.	Gandalf (*Lord of the Rings*)
Kind aunt, sibling, cousin	James Bond	Dalai Lama
Best friend	Gladiator	Nelson Mandela
Pet dog/cat	Partner, best friend, sibling	God
Florence Nightingale/ nurse	Police officer	Dumbledore (*Harry Potter*)
Mary Poppins	Aragorn (*Lord of the Rings*)	Wise Owl
Character from movie or book	Aslan (*Narnia*)	Socrates
Jesus	Panther/Lion/Bear	Galadriel (*Lord of the Rings*)
Partner, if good relationship	Angel	King Solomon

For this exercise you may like to pick one for each category. The character or animal should embody the relevant characteristic of compassion, strength or wisdom to guide you if you don't know what to do. This exercise is very similar to the Safe Place.

Bring your chosen Compassionate character to mind and imagine them alongside you to provide love and comfort. Whilst butterfly tapping very slowly, focus on their physical features, the expression in their eyes, the colour of their hair or fur. Then notice the sound of their voice. Hear what you want them to say to you. Continue on with imagining the way you want them to relate to you specifically, i.e. do you want an arm around you? Imagine the compassion and love flowing from them towards you and stay with the way this feels, slowly butterfly tapping all the time. This can be a very moving exercise.

For Protection, you can equip your character with whatever you want them to have, so be creative. They may have swords, shields or superpowers! Do exactly the same as with the Compassionate figure by imagining them alongside you, to protect you; focus on what you see, hear and feel whilst slowly butterfly tapping all the time.

For Wisdom, this is somebody who can help you to solve an impossible situation. Go through the same as above, focusing on them being able to guide you as you connect with feeling them alongside you.

Subject Index

Author Index